D1409090

Transitions in Care

Meeting the Challenges of Type 1 Diabetes in Young Adults

Howard A. Wolpert, MD
Barbara J. Anderson, PhD
Jill Weissberg-Benchell, PhD, CDE

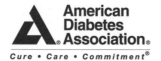

American Diabetes Association.

Cure • Care • Commitment®

Director, Book Publishing, Robert Anthony; *Managing Editor,* Abe Ogden; *Acquisitions Editor, Professional Books,* Victor Van Beuren; *Editor,* Wendy M. Martin; *Production Manager,* Melissa Sprott; *Composition,* Circle Graphics; *Cover Design,* Koncept, Inc.; *Printer,* Victor Graphics.

Printed in the United States of America
1 3 5 7 9 10 8 6 4 2

The suggestions and information contained in this publication are generally consistent with the *Clinical Practice Recommendations* and other policies of the American Diabetes Association, but they do not represent the policy or position of the Association or any of its boards or committees. Reasonable steps have been taken to ensure the accuracy of the information presented. However, the American Diabetes Association cannot ensure the safety or efficacy of any product or service described in this publication. Individuals are advised to consult a physician or other appropriate health care professional before undertaking any diet or exercise program or taking any medication referred to in this publication. Professionals must use and apply their own professional judgment, experience, and training and should not rely solely on the information contained in this publication before prescribing any diet, exercise, or medication. The American Diabetes Association— its officers, directors, employees, volunteers, and members—assumes no responsibility or liability for personal or other injury, loss, or damage that may result from the suggestions or information in this publication.

⊚ The paper in this publication meets the requirements of the ANSI Standard Z39.48-1992 (permanence of paper).

ADA titles may be purchased for business or promotional use or for special sales. To purchase more than 50 copies of this book at a discount, or for custom editions of this book with your logo, contact the American Diabetes Association at the address below, at booksales@diabetes.org, or by calling 703-299-2046.

American Diabetes Association
1701 North Beauregard Street
Alexandria, Virginia 22311

DOI: 10.2337/9781580403245

Library of Congress Cataloging-in-Publication Data

Wolpert, Howard, 1958-
Transitions in care : a guide on the challenges of type 1 diabetes in the young adult period for patients, their families, and health care providers / Howard A. Wolpert, Barbara J. Anderson, Jill Weissberg-Benchell.
     p. ; cm.
Includes bibliographical references and index.
ISBN 978-1-58040-324-5 (alk. paper)
1. Diabetes in youth. 2. Diabetes in adolescence. I. Anderson, Barbara J. (Barbara Jane), 1947- II. Weissberg-Benchell, Jill. III. American Diabetes Association. IV. Title.
[DNLM: 1. Diabetes Mellitus, Type 1. 2. Young Adult. 3. Adolescent. WK 810 W866ta 2009]

RJ420.D5W65 2009
616.4'6200835--dc22
                                    2008050822

Contents

III

For Parents: Helping Your Child During the Transition to Young Adulthood   59

IV

Clinical Principles for the Health Care Professional 71

Prelude: Why We Wrote This Book

Almost anyone who has cared for someone in their late teens and 20s, through either parenting or treatment, knows that this is a unique and distinct phase of life. These are times filled with the tasks that map out the course of a life: the engrossing search for self and one's place in society, the first steps toward career and financial independence, and deepening emotional involvements. The young adult is no longer an adolescent, but frequently is not yet completely independent from family support either. This is also a time of life when the person with type 1 diabetes assumes full responsibility for his or her own diabetes care and a period when the earliest signs of diabetes complications will often first present. The initiation of intensive therapy during this phase, when lifelong patterns of self-care behavior are being set, can have a significant impact on an individual's risk for future complications.

Intensive insulin therapy requires discipline and sacrifice, not to mention responsibility and adequate support. Clearly, for the young adult who faces many competing demands for his or her time and attention, diabetes self-care may not always be a priority. The diabetes clinician needs to be aware that any perceived reluctance to intensify therapy on the part of the young adult patient may be because his or her focus is naturally drawn to the competing demands of education, relationships, and career-building. A successful relationship with a diabetes clinician will be founded in a long-term view of care, focusing primarily on a directly collaborative partnership that ensures that the young adult remains actively involved in his or her own health care. Clinicians can jump-start this process by envisioning their primary role as an agent for behavioral change. The clinician's role should resemble that of a *coach* (who equips young adults with the skills needed to manage their diabetes) and a *guide* (who helps young adults make informed decisions about living with diabetes and works with the patient in developing a plan aimed at reaching optimal diabetes control). A priority in care is to ensure that patients remain invested in their self-care behaviors and engage in active problem-solving. Young adults who have these tools are less likely to fall into the trap of frustration, hopelessness, and disengagement from medical follow-up.

We have found that the needs of young adults with diabetes fall outside of the traditional focus of both adult and pediatric medicine; that is the reason for this book. Our clinical experience has taught us the importance of a thoughtful, systematic approach to assist young adults in their transition to healthy adulthood. In this book, we offer a framework for thinking about the important issues in diabetes care for young adults. The first section provides background information on the young adult period with which young adults with diabetes, their parents, and care providers should be familiar. After that, the book is written in two voices. One voice, introduced in the second and third sections and directed to young adults and their families and friends, focuses on the challenges and demands of living with diabetes and presents guidance in making informed individual and family decisions about diabetes management during this complex phase of life. The other voice, arising in the fourth section, provides a perspective on how the complexities of this developmental stage affect the health professional's clinical role.

Although we have used different voices for each section, this hardly means that each part of the book is exclusive to that audience. We strongly encourage you, whether you are a young adult, parent, or care provider, to cover all of this material. Knowledge, particularly when concerning diabetes, is one of the most important tools in optimizing care, especially for a patient group that has been largely overlooked in clinical history.

Howard A. Wolpert, MD
Joslin Diabetes Center, Boston, MA
Barbara J. Anderson, PhD
Baylor College of Medicine, Houston, TX
Jill Weissberg-Benchell, PhD, CDE
Children's Memorial Hospital, Chicago, IL

The Challenges of Young Adulthood

DEVELOPMENTAL ISSUES IN THE YOUNG ADULT (EMERGING ADULTHOOD)

Over the past century, traditional developmental psychology theorists such as Erik Erikson (1950, 1968) defined the time immediately after adolescence as the "young adult period." In contrast, J. J. Arnett (2000, 2004), a leading contemporary developmental theorist, argued that young adulthood does not begin until youths are in their late 20s or 30s and that the developmental stage between approximately 18 and 25 years defines a period called "emerging adulthood." Recent cultural trends in America for young people in their 20s lead them to delay assuming adult roles with respect to marriage, parenting, and work. Arnett suggests that today's young people should:

"... *explore the possibilities available to them in love and work, and move gradually toward making enduring choices. . . . This period is a time of high hopes and big dreams. However, it is also a time of anxiety and uncertainty, because the lives of young people are so unsettled, and many of them have no idea where their explorations will lead. They struggle with uncertainty even as they revel in being freer than they ever were in childhood or ever will be once they take on the full weight of adult responsibilities. To be a young American today is to experience both excitement and uncertainty, wide-open possibility and confusion, new freedoms, and new fears.*" (Arnett 2004)

Furthermore, in contrast to the views of traditional developmental psychology, more recent developmental theorists subdivide the young adult or post-adolescent period into two phases: an early phase corresponding to the years after high school (~18–22 years of age) and a later phase when more traditional adult roles are assumed (~23–30 years of age). This age division is somewhat arbitrary and may not apply to all individuals, and not all individuals or cultures progress through the young adult period according to these two phases. However, thinking about young adulthood as consisting of two phases provides a valuable framework when considering diabetes management and may help to ensure that the clinician's approach and focus is appropriately matched to the young adult's life circumstances and readiness to become an active participant in his or her own diabetes management.

THE FIRST PHASE OF THE YOUNG ADULT PERIOD

Levinson et al. (1978) and Arnett (2004) theorized that, in the U.S., there is frequently a misfit between the developmental tasks of young adults just after high school and the expectations of the various institutions responsible for young adults. Arnett studied individuals between the ages of 18 and 24 years and asked them what attributes made someone an adult. Four specific achievements were cited: *1)* the ability to accept responsibility for oneself, *2)* the ability to make independent decisions, *3)* the ability to become financially independent, and *4)* the ability to independently form one's own beliefs and values. Interestingly, most of the young adults interviewed did not believe that they had achieved these goals. In fact, the majority of young people in the U.S. do not believe that they have achieved these goals until they are in their late 20s.

Several dilemmas confront patients in the first phase of the young adult period. This phase brings desire for independence, yet also fear of independence. Freedom from parental supervision and rules also brings responsibilities than can be quite daunting. The young adult begins to face issues such as, how do you find/keep a place to live, pay your bills, balance a checkbook, manage credit, begin a relationship/keep a relationship that might be "forever," and choose a career? While young adults are trying to balance all of these new freedoms and responsibilities, they are probably doing this with less help from their parents and less structure in their daily routine. In addition, if young adults have moved away from their hometown, they are making these decisions in a place where few people know them, often removed from their closest friends. Arnett suggests that individuals in this first phase are beginning to "explore the possibilities available to them in love and work and move gradually toward making enduring choices." He suggests these actions might lead them to feel unsettled, since they do not yet know where these explorations will lead them.

Similarly, the young adult's family faces several dilemmas as the family begins to address issues such as the following:

- Whether the young adult and his or her parents tolerate the separation and increasing independence and still remain connected.
- Whether the parents become over-involved or cut off relationships prematurely.
- How young adults cope with the potential of remaining dependent on their parents for both tangible (e.g., monetary, housing) and emotional support as they develop their skills and identities as either students or workers.
- How the possibility of financial dependence affects the relationship between the young adult and his or her parents and the parents' ability to treat their older children as adults with separate, independent lives.
- How parents cope with the difficult transition from a hands-on role in the care of their child to being a "consultant." Similarly, the shift from speaking directly to their child's physician or nurse to now relying on secondhand (if any) information is a transition that raises most parents' anxiety and concern.

To place the dilemmas young adults and their families face in perspective, the data from the 2000 Census tell us that 56% of men and 43% of women between the ages of 18 and 24 years still live at home with their parents. Moreover, 30% of men and 35% of women in that age-group live with roommates. In fact, only 4% of individuals in this age-group live alone. Therefore, the assumption that individuals in this age-group are independent may be false, both from a theoretical perspective on adult development and also from a fact-based perspective regarding where and with whom they live.

During the early phase of young adulthood, which Levinson et al. (1978) called the "early adult transition," the person may be transitioning geographically, economically, and emotionally away from the parental home. Furthermore, if the 18- to 22-year-old young adult has also transitioned to a college or trade school, his or her new life will be marked by added changes, distractions, and demands. For most young adults, these competing educational, economic, and social priorities detract from a focused commitment to chronic disease management. Even though young adults are facing these competing demands, most do not believe that they have achieved all of the skills necessary to remain independent and accept these responsibilities on their own. Therefore, it may be unrealistic to expect young adults with diabetes in this first phase of young adulthood to intensify their glycemic control, to learn pump therapy, or even to transition to a new adult diabetes provider. Furthermore, for most patients, this early phase is often marked by feelings of invulnerability and a tendency to reject perceptions of adult control, and this further limits receptiveness to change.

Lessons from Psychosocial Research in Youth with Type 1 Diabetes After Adolescence

Emerging adults with diabetes face even more complicated decisions than their healthy peers. The daily demands of diabetes care (which include the need to coordinate daily care, finding appropriate care providers, and the daunting task of access to appropriate supplies and medical care) must be woven into all of the normative choices regarding relationships, occupations, living arrangements, and financial management. The following review of empirical behavioral studies of post-adolescent youth with type 1 diabetes illustrates two ideas central to this discussion: *1*) the developmental period after high school represents a distinct period with unique demands separate from adolescence and *2*) for a subgroup of young adults, there is continuity between the diabetes-specific adherence and control problems they experienced as adolescents and the ongoing adherence behavior and glycemic control struggles they face over the post-adolescent years. The earliest psychosocial studies of post-adolescent youth (18- to 25-year-old individuals) with type 1 diabetes suggested that these individuals experienced a delay in psychosocial maturation (Jacobson et al. 1982, Kokkonen et al. 1997, Robinson et al. 1989, Kokkonen et al. 1994, Myers 1997). It is important to remember that the majority of patients on whom these empirical studies were based experienced their childhood and adolescent years with diabetes during the period before the Diabetes Control and Complications Trial

(DCCT) (i.e., before the era of intensive management of type 1 diabetes with the added burden of a more complex treatment regimen that allows for more lifestyle flexibility).

More recent empirical studies, carried out in the post-DCCT era, have reported findings that contradict these earlier reports of delayed psychosocial maturation in post-adolescent youth with type 1 diabetes. Pacaud et al. (2007) in Canada studied the psychosocial maturation of individuals 18–25 years of age with type 1 diabetes and age-matched control subjects who did not have diabetes. The mean age of respondents in both groups was 22 years of age. The authors concluded that the youth with type 1 diabetes did not differ from healthy peers in terms of psychosocial maturation. Interestingly, there was a tendency for respondents in both groups to score lower than the norms on indexes of responsibility and independence. This study supports Arnett's theory that it is not until their late 20s that many youth in today's world begin to assume traditionally more "adult" roles (Arnett 2004). Similarly, Gillibrand and Stevenson (2006) recently studied young people 16–25 years old with type 1 diabetes living in the U.K. and also found that emerging adults with diabetes have normal levels of psychosocial maturation. Of great importance, and a theme that is woven throughout this book, Gillibrand and Stevenson (2006) also found that a high level of family support during this key developmental phase was the strongest predictor of the young adult's adherence to the diabetes regimen.

Whereas the cross-sectional studies of Pacaud et al. (2007) and Gillibrand and Stevenson (2006) documented normal psychosocial maturation for young adults with type 1 diabetes, the longitudinal cohort research of Bryden and colleagues in the U.K. identified a subgroup of young adults with disordered eating (insulin misuse for weight management), especially in female adolescents with type 1 diabetes. This disordered eating was strongly related to the development of microvascular complications and mortality among the young adult females in this cohort (Bryden et al. 1999, Peveler et al. 2005). This 8-year follow-up study of a cohort of adolescents with diabetes found that behavioral problems during the adolescent years predicted poorer glycemic control in young adulthood and a significant increase in serious microvascular complications. During the follow-up evaluation of these individuals, 54% of the young adult females were overweight (BMI >25.0 kg/m^2), up from 21% at baseline. This weight gain can be an important factor contributing to poor ongoing diabetes self-management and adherence.

Over 35% of adolescents and young adult females with type 1 diabetes in the U.K. acknowledged intentional reduction or omission of insulin to control weight (Peveler et al. 2005). Rydall et al. (1997) also followed a group of adolescent females with type 1 diabetes and found high rates of microvascular complications in the young women with disordered eating behavior. Consistent with the findings from the U.K., Goebel-Fabbri et al. (2008) from the U.S. followed an initial sample of 390 women with type 1 diabetes, 30% of whom had admitted to restricting insulin to lose weight. Eleven years later, 234 of the original participants were reached. Findings suggest that insulin restriction conveyed a three-fold increased risk of death, underscoring the potential dangers inherent in disordered eating among individuals with diabetes.

Concerns about weight management and the potentially dangerous strategies youths with diabetes may use to achieve weight-related goals cannot be understated. Findings from the 8-year prospective study previously mentioned by Bryden et al. (1999, 2001) revealed that glycemic control was the worst for the disordered eating subgroup in late adolescence, especially in females. In the Peveler study (2005), the proportion of individuals who were overweight increased for both males and females. A quarter of the male patients and over one-third of females developed complications, and these patients had significantly higher mean A1C levels than those young adults without complications. Psychological and behavioral problems at baseline were related to higher A1C levels across the 8-year study period, indicating that behavioral problems in adolescence significantly influenced glycemic control during the young adult period (Bryden et al. 2001).

Similar conclusions about the continuity of adherence and glycemic control problems over the late-adolescent/early-adult years have been reported by Wysocki et al. (1992) in a cross-sectional study of 18- to 22-year-old youth with type 1 diabetes. Subsequently, Bryden et al. (2003) published a report that followed a group of young adults 17–25 years of age over an 11-year period into adulthood. There was no improvement in glycemic control over this period. The proportion of patients having serious complications increased over this period, and females were more likely than males to have multiple diabetes complications. Psychiatric symptoms in late adolescence and young adulthood predicted psychiatric problems later in the cohort.

In summary, the most recent psychosocial research has documented that the majority of post-adolescent youth with type 1 diabetes in the post-DCCT era do not demonstrate delays in psychosocial maturity. However, studies have documented that post-adolescent patients have specialized needs with respect to their diabetes care during the vulnerable and transitional period after high school. Moreover, there is a subgroup of adolescent patients with type 1 diabetes, especially females, who are at an increased risk for the downward cycle of mental health problems (especially disordered eating behaviors and diagnosable eating disorders), poor glycemic control, and the development of microvascular complications of type 1 diabetes. Longitudinal follow-up studies of adolescent patients have indicated that for this subgroup of youth at high risk for the interrelated problems of poor control, psychiatric problems, and diabetes complications, these problems only worsen over the late adolescent and "emerging adulthood" years. Therefore, whether you are a person with diabetes, the parent of someone with diabetes, or a diabetes care provider, if you are concerned about eating issues, weight issues, or other potential emotional and behavioral issues that are known to affect diabetes self-care, please discuss these concerns openly and seek appropriate support from friends, family, colleagues, and mental health professionals.

Issues That Affect the Transition of Care for Adolescents with Type 1 Diabetes

The length of time the young adult has had diabetes can be an important factor in the transition of the young adult to independent self-management. For some young adults who have had diabetes since childhood, it is important to explore formative diabetes experiences. Longitudinal studies of pediatric patients with type 1 diabetes in the U.K. and U.S. have reported that behavior problems during the adolescent years clearly predict emotional and physical health complications in the young adult period. The young adult who as a child faced unrealistic expectations for self-care behavior and glucose control and had a legacy of punitive and judgmental medical encounters is especially vulnerable to "diabetes burnout," a condition characterized by feelings of inadequacy or guilt from chronically failing at diabetes management.

If the young adult has had a negative socialization experience growing up with diabetes and does not have a solid, constructive relationship with pediatric providers, early transfer to an adult provider (having some experience with adolescents and young adults with type 1 diabetes) may

STEVE'S STORY: The Impact of Negative Feedback

Steve T., a 22-year-old college senior at the University of Texas, originally from New Jersey, was diagnosed with type 1 diabetes when he was 8 years old. Steve has not seen a diabetes clinician during the 4 years he has been in college in Texas. He is an engineering major and is now looking for jobs after he graduates. Steve is on a regimen of two injections a day and has not monitored his blood glucose at all during college. For the first time, Steve is having frequent "insulin reactions" as he is beginning his job search. Therefore, Steve decides to see a doctor in Texas for his diabetes. When he meets with the diabetes team, he reports that he takes two shots a day, does not change his insulin dose, and does not check his blood glucose levels. When the educator tells him that his A1C is 10% and that he needs to check his blood glucose to adjust his insulin dose, Steve says, "Just tell me how much more insulin to give. I don't want to get back into that horrible grind of checking my blood sugars." Steve reports that his diabetes team in New Jersey made him feel that he could never get his A1C or his daily blood glucose in the "right range," although he monitored his glucose three to four times each day in high school. And he reports that his parents always criticized his blood glucose numbers, convinced that he was sneaking all of the wrong foods behind their backs. In fact, they took away the keys to his car if he had a lot of blood glucose levels that were not in the right range. Steve's experiences as a teenager monitoring his blood glucose were so negative that he feels he cannot face the possibility of monitoring his glucose levels again. For Steve, blood glucose monitoring led to feedback that was blaming, threatening, and demoralizing. Steve has diabetes burnout.

be in the patient's best interest. One program for post-adolescent youth with type 1 diabetes was reported by Van Walleghem et al. (2006). This study assessed the feasibility and acceptability of an innovative transition service initiated to serve 18- to 30-year-old subjects with type 1 diabetes as they transitioned between pediatric and adult care in Manitoba, Canada. The "maestro" service identified and coordinated access to appropriate support services in the community for young adults with type 1 diabetes. The maestro or "health navigator" was an administrative coordinator who maintained telephone and e-mail contact with the young adults to help them identify barriers to accessing appropriate adult health care services. A comprehensive array of communication channels was established: a website; a bimonthly newsletter; drop-in, informal patient educational dinner events; and patient discussion/support groups. Over the first two and a half years of the project, 79% of eligible patients participated in the program, requesting assistance for both access to care and educational programs. In addition, results indicated that this model of service was feasible and acceptable for young adults with type 1 diabetes as they transition from pediatric to adult care.

The maestro program's focus on improved communication was an important key to their success, as concerns about poor communication between families and providers have been noted as barriers to successful transitions. Two large population-based surveys of youths receiving medical care for a variety of conditions, with sample sizes of at least 4,000 in each study (Lotstein et al. 2005, Scal and Ireland 2005), found that only half of the parents talked about transition issues with their child's physician, and of those who did discuss these issues, only 30–42% discussed shifting care to an adult provider. Similarly, adolescents do not feel that they receive adequate information regarding transition issues (Telfair et al. 2004), and they worry about leaving their familiar health care team for an unknown medical provider. In a study in youth with diabetes, Eiser et al. (1993) found that youths conceptualized pediatric programs as family-centered, informal, and socially oriented. In contrast, they conceptualized adult programs as more formal, with an emphasis on the risks of long-term complications. Dovey-Pearce et al. (2005) found that youth with diabetes want to work with clinicians who try to integrate their life circumstances into recommendations for diabetes care.

The need for improved communication and information sharing when fostering successful transitions was underscored by studies conducted by Pacaud et al. (1996, 2005). These authors surveyed patients with diabetes who had been transferred from a pediatric program to an adult program. The first survey occurred in Montreal and the second (almost 10 years later) occurred in Alberta. The findings from these surveys were the same: 31% of the adolescents had a lapse of over 6 months between their last pediatric visit and their first adult visit, with 11% lost to follow-up. Young adults expressed the belief that their transition was abrupt, that they lacked information about resources, and that it was difficult to coordinate all of the subspecialties they needed to see (e.g., endocrinologist, dietitian). Similarly, Kipps et al. (2002) assessed patient perceptions regarding transition experiences for 229 youth with diabetes. Although 90% transitioned to adult services at 17 years of age, only 61% regularly attended an adult care program 2 years after transfer.

Some patients will transition easily. Others may benefit from continuing to follow up with familiar pediatric providers and educators during the vulnerable post–high school period and delay transition to adult care until the distractions and insecurities of this period have passed. Discussions about transition issues during the early adolescent years among all of the interested parties (patient, parent, provider) will likely help. In addition, establishing effective means of communication and scheduling a meeting with the adult provider before making the transition (Brumfield and Lansbury 2004) seem to increase the likelihood of success. Finally, longitudinal research by Bryden and colleagues suggests that teens who display behavioral difficulties during adolescence experience poorer glycemic control as young adults. Therefore, openly discussing past emotional and behavioral issues is also an important goal in transition planning.

THE SECOND PHASE OF THE YOUNG ADULT PERIOD

During the second phase of the young adult period (typically between 23 and 30 years of age), there is often a maturing sense of identity and more "adult-like" roles in society, such as a stable intimate relationship, employment, and financial independence. This phase, when the individual starts making plans about his or her future life, is usually accompanied by a growing recognition of the importance of striving for better glycemic control and a receptiveness to improving self-care behavior. Life partners can be important supports and agents for change, and a shared sense of investment in the future will often catalyze this change in self-care behavior. This period (when lifelong patterns of behavior are set) can be a critical "window of opportunity" for health care and educational interventions. Health care providers and educators have a crucial role at this stage in preparing and motivating the young adult with diabetes to assume self-management responsibilities.

JIM'S STORY: Finding a Diabetes Team That Fits Your Lifestyle

Jim is a 27-year-old young man who has had diabetes since age 11. Jim's parents were very involved in diabetes management throughout his adolescence, and his father followed a structured daily exercise routine and meal plan just like Jim's to provide support. Jim went to college in his hometown and lived at home. During this time, his parents maintained their support and structured routines for diabetes care. After college, Jim moved away to New York City for a job opportunity in the financial area, and he got very caught up in the fast-paced banking world in which he worked. However, he was not able to maintain his strict approach to eating and exercise with his new lifestyle in New York City. His new peers ate out for most meals and the portion sizes were considerably larger than he was used to. He became very depressed about not exercising and about overeating, and he steadily gained weight. Jim was feeling discouraged about his diabetes management, and for the first time, he felt it was too much to handle. The turning point in his thinking about diabetes self-care came when he decided to enter law school and met a young woman there and became engaged. With her encouragement, Jim finally sought out a new diabetes team in New York City, and his educator and doctor introduced him to the idea of carbohydrate counting and multiple daily insulin injections, which allowed him to have a more flexible lifestyle that fit his work and life in New York City.

PART Two

Getting Prepared for Your Journey with Diabetes through Young Adulthood

YOU DON'T NEED A SERMON, BUT THE BASICS WON'T HURT

There's a good chance that from the minute you were diagnosed with diabetes, you've been overwhelmed with the same message: Get your blood glucose under control and your chances for a long, complication-free life will dramatically increase. We could give you examples, such as the DCCT, where over 1,400 individuals with diabetes were divided into two groups: a "conventional" group that took up to two insulin injections a day (which was the usual standard of care at the time the study was started in the 1980s) and an "intensive" group that used multiple injections or an insulin pump. As you probably already guessed, the intensive group ended up in a lot better shape. In fact, they had less than half as many severe eye, kidney, and nerve complications as people in the conventional group.

But you probably already knew this. Maybe not specifically, but you had a good idea that better blood glucose control means healthier living. So you don't need any more sermons from health professionals! You know *why* you should strive to have the best glucose control possible. The challenge is *how* you achieve good control and *how* you balance the day-to-day demands of diabetes with the other demands (and pleasures!) of life. In this section, we will explore this difficult balancing act between diabetes and the rest of your life. In addition, we will outline a roadmap, which may help you get and stay on track with your diabetes.

UNDERSTANDING INSULIN REPLACEMENT

Before we get to the principles about how to achieve good blood glucose control, we're going to present a brief review of how insulin regulates glucose metabolism in the body. As you probably know, insulin is a hormone produced by the beta-cells in the pancreas. There are two different components to the insulin in circulation (see Figure 1):

- Background insulin (also commonly referred to as *basal* insulin) controls the blood glucose levels in between meals and overnight. During these periods, the liver (which acts like the body's glucose reservoir) is continuously releasing glucose into the bloodstream to provide energy for basic functions in the body. Insulin helps control this process. Without basal insulin, there would be an excessive release of glucose by the liver, and glucose levels in the blood would rise. In addition, in the absence of basal insulin, the liver starts producing ketone bodies, and these can accumulate in the blood, leading to a dangerous condition known as *diabetic ketoacidosis.*
- Insulin surges at mealtimes (also commonly referred to as insulin *boluses*) cause the tissues of the body to take up glucose from the bloodstream. The amount of insulin produced in these mealtime surges is precisely controlled to ensure that there is just enough to take care of the carbohydrates being eaten. Eat a bit more, and more insulin is produced; eat a bit less, and less insulin is produced.

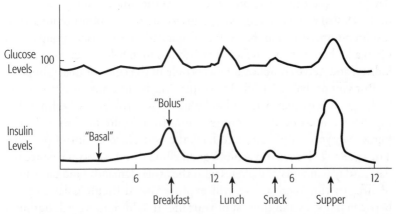

FIGURE 1 A 24-hour insulin and glucose profile in a person without diabetes.

In type 1 diabetes, the immune system (which is normally involved in combating infections) misguidedly attacks and destroys the beta-cells in the pancreas. The end result is that the body can no longer produce insulin. The fundamental challenge in treating type 1 diabetes is in replacing the insulin your body is no longer making and taking just enough insulin to match your body's needs. Too much insulin leads to low blood glucose levels and too little leads to high blood glucose. Trying to avoid large ups and downs in your glucose numbers is another challenge in treating type 1 diabetes; dramatic variations in your numbers can be particularly unpleasant.

APPROACHES TO INSULIN TREATMENT

The insulin profile shown in Figure 2 may be familiar to you. In this traditional approach to insulin replacement, there are two injections of rapid-acting insulin (Apidra, Humalog, Novolog, or regular) at breakfast and dinner and two injections of a longer-acting insulin (NPH) to provide your body with basal insulin. Typically, the rapid-acting and longer-acting insulins are either premixed in one vial or one pen, or you can mix the two insulins into one syringe, so that you administer two

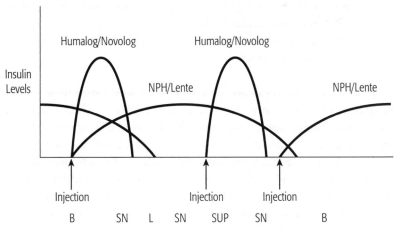

FIGURE 2 Injection therapy using Humalog/Novolog and NPH/lente. In this approach, there are two injections of rapid-acting insulin at breakfast and dinner and two injections of NPH/lente insulin to provide the basal insulin. B, breakfast; L, lunch; SN, snack; SUP, supper.

injections per day, with two different insulins in each injection. The rapid-acting insulin injections take care of the carbohydrates eaten at breakfast and dinner, while the morning injection of NPH covers lunch and the evening injection of NPH controls the sugar that the liver releases into the bloodstream overnight. Striving for good glucose control using this type of insulin program can be challenging. These are some of the constraints:

- If lunch is delayed, the morning injection of NPH will kick in and hypoglycemia (low blood glucose reaction) could result.
- Snacks will often need to be eaten between meals (especially midmorning and bedtime) to prevent the long-acting insulin from causing hypoglycemia.
- Lunch and snacks will need to have a consistent carbohydrate content. If you eat too many carbohydrates, there may be insufficient insulin in the system and the blood glucose level will end up rising. If you eat too few carbohydrates, there may be more insulin in your body than you need to cover your food, and your blood glucose level may fall.
- Waking times in the morning need to be consistent from one day to the next. If you get up later in the morning, the longer-acting insulin taken the evening before (to control the production of glucose by the liver overnight) may be running out, and the end result will be an increased glucose level.
- Hypoglycemia in the middle of the night can occur if a bedtime snack is not consumed.

As with most choices in our lives, there is a tradeoff with these insulin programs. There is no need for a lunchtime injection, which can be an important consideration for someone who would find this extra injection inconvenient or impractical at school. But if you want to keep your glucose levels within any targeted range, you need to follow a fairly regimented and consistent routine and meal plan. This means that meals and snacks need to be eaten at specific times, and the carbohydrate content of meals needs to be consistent from one day to the next. To address the risk of hypoglycemia in the middle of the night, some people will administer the rapid-acting insulin at dinner and the longer-acting insulin at bedtime. That way, the NPH is not peaking at 2:00 a.m. when you are asleep. This choice of an insulin regimen means administering three injections per day.

The development of peakless long-acting insulins and insulin pumps has presented new options for insulin replacement. With these tools, we can be closer to mimicking the way the beta-cells of the pancreas release insulin into the body.

This approach to insulin replacement (shown in Figure 3)—also known as *basal/bolus therapy*—allows more flexibility in a person's schedule and eating. Insulin can be matched to cover the amount of food eaten, and there's no need to eat on schedule. In addition, because the longer-acting insulin does not peak, there is no need to eat snacks between meals to prevent hypoglycemia. This can be quite helpful with weight control (see page 32). But this type of insulin program generally requires more injections per day or the use of an insulin pump.

DECIDING WHICH INSULIN PROGRAM IS RIGHT FOR YOU

Some individuals will need a different insulin program for each phase of their life. For example, during the school years, when taking a lunchtime injection in the cafeteria can be impractical, the NPH-based insulin program may work best. Later during the college years, the extra flexibility provided by the basal/bolus program may be a real advantage. There are a couple of considerations in weighing the decision about whether to use injections or a pump for basal/bolus insulin replacement. Some find

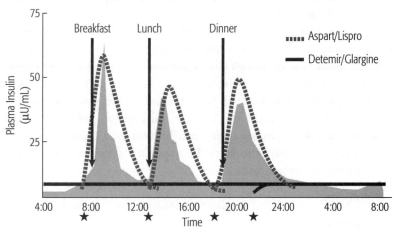

FIGURE 3 Schematic showing basal insulin (glargine or determir) and mealtime rapid-acting insulin such as aspart, lispro, and glulisine.

that it can be a hassle to take an extra injection every time they want to snack or have eaten more than planned, and with a pump, it is easy to take a bolus of insulin whenever there is a need. However, before you decide on the pump, there are two key questions you should ask yourself. First, "How comfortable will I be with wearing a pump and having an outward sign of diabetes?" and second, "Do I have enough time to attend to the extra demands of using a pump?" The early adult and college years are often a time when serious relationships (both romantic and platonic) outside of the family first develop, and some people will find the pump a bit too obvious and public. The added responsibility of starting pump therapy can be too much to handle if you have a lot of other commitments in your life. Some find it's better to deal with the demands of getting settled into a new job or college before trying the pump. Because it is you who lives with and manages your diabetes day-to-day, only you will really know which type of insulin program will suit you best. The decision should be yours—made in consultation with your health care provider.

FUNDAMENTAL SKILLS IN MANAGING DIABETES

You have probably already discovered that the key skill in managing your diabetes is in *learning how to think like a pancreas*—understanding how to match up insulin with the carbohydrates you eat. Therefore, the essential elements in learning how to regulate your diabetes are having an understanding of how insulin acts and knowing the carbohydrate content of your foods.

A comprehensive review of all the knowledge needed to tighten up glucose control is beyond the scope of this book. However, as you are moving toward the post–high school phase of your life, there are a number of important skills and concepts that you need to master. Look at the list we offer below and see if you feel comfortable in your knowledge of these topics. If not, use this outline as discussion points with your diabetes team when you see them next. This can be a great opportunity to advocate for yourself. Some of the important skills you will need to master include the following:

- Understanding how the different insulins you take peak and act in your body.
- Learning about the carbohydrate and fat content of the foods in your diet. This includes learning how to read food labels (and which

Pros and Cons of Pump Therapy

Pros:
- Greater lifestyle flexibility and freedom
- Greater sense of control over diabetes
- Greater sense of well-being from a reduction in glucose fluctuations
- Promise of a healthier future
- Help with the dawn phenomenon (increased release of glucose by the liver during the early morning ["dawn"] period)
- Improved ability to recognize low blood glucose reactions (see Bumps in the Journey: Intensive Therapy and Hypoglycemia on page 24)
- Improved control during physical activity
- Easier weight control (see More Bumps in the Journey: Intensive Therapy and Weight Gain on page 32)

Cons:
- Pumps are a visible sign of diabetes
- Extra time and effort required to get started and use the pump
- Inconvenient to wear
- Increased risk for diabetic ketoacidosis
- Must monitor blood glucose at least four times a day
- Added responsibility of taking care of the catheter sites and pump
- Extra troubleshooting skills required
- Catheter site infection
- Cost

For more information to help you decide whether the pump is right for you, see *Smart Pumping for People with Diabetes: A Practical Approach to Mastering the Insulin Pump* (Wolpert 2002).

parts of the food labels are most important) and judge portion sizes. Sometimes keeping a food diary can be helpful.
- Using blood glucose monitoring to decide about insulin doses and using the numbers from your logbooks to identify glucose patterns.
- Learning how to troubleshoot and treat hypoglycemia (low blood glucose reactions).

- Learning how physical activity affects glucose control and how to regulate your glucose levels during and after exercise (see Getting Physical on page 54).
- Learning how to manage your diabetes during illness and sick-days.
- Learning how alcohol affects your glucose control and how to manage your diabetes when you drink (see page 52).

This learning will be an ongoing lifelong process, and as you progress further, you will find that that there will always be some additional information or insights that can be important to you. For example, the fat in your diet (sometimes hidden in muffins, pizza, and fries) can make your body less responsive (sensitive) to insulin and can also have a big impact on your blood glucose after meals. So this may be something you will also need to pay attention to as you progress in optimizing your glucose control. Figure 4 illustrates some of the factors that affect the delicate balance between high and low glucose levels.

For more information on intensive insulin and pump therapy, see the *Complete Guide to Diabetes* (American Diabetes Association 2005). Your state chapter of the American Diabetes Association (ADA) can put you

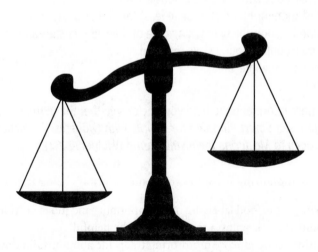

Insulin & Exercise: Food & Stress:
Decrease glucose levels   Increase glucose levels

FIGURE 4 The balance between high and low glucose levels.

in touch with ADA-recognized education programs that offer guidance and instruction in diabetes self-management.

KEEPING PERSPECTIVE ABOUT MONITORING AND NUMBERS

As already mentioned, expanding your knowledge base and developing a sense of mastery of how all of these factors (insulin, food, exercise, etc.) affect your blood glucose level can take years of experience. Remember that despite the recent advances in the development of new insulins, pumps, and monitoring devices, the tools we have to manage type 1 diabetes today are still imperfect. There is no magic formula for getting perfect glucose numbers. No one living with diabetes can always keep their blood glucose numbers between 80 and 120. Having consistently perfect numbers is an unattainable goal—and so is being a Nobel laureate before the age of 30, or running a mile in under 3 minutes, or shooting a 50 in an 18-hole game of golf. Setting goals that are out of reach will likely cause frustration. There may be some periods in life, such as during pregnancy, where one's energies and priorities are focused on ensuring remarkably tight glucose control. However, it is usually difficult for women to sustain these tight goals once the pregnancy is over and attention is focused on the needs of the newborn and the other demands of life.

Having realistic goals is the key to living well with diabetes and to living well in all aspects of your life. It is also important to keep in mind that if your personal blood glucose goal is 70–180 mg/dl, you should aim for the *average* of your blood glucose measurements to be in that range. This does *not* necessarily mean that all (or even most) of your individual measurements will be in that target range. The object of monitoring is not to "test" your performance; it's to give you the information you need for the daily management of diabetes and to identify glucose trends that will be helpful in optimizing your treatment. It can become demoralizing if your performance is always being tested, so try to avoid viewing glucose monitoring as a test. Instead, try to think of your glucose monitoring (or "checks") as a compass that gives you direction ("How much insulin do I need?" "Is it safe to drive?" "Do I still need to continue snacking to treat my low?").

Also keep in mind that just because there is no way to achieve perfect numbers, it does not mean that you should give up trying to do your best. You actually have control over a great many aspects of your diabetes care, and the things you can control can make a huge difference in how you feel today and in your future health. Developing a sense of confidence that you have some control over blood glucose levels can come quickly, but this needs to be balanced with an appreciation that our bodies do not always respond as anticipated. Even individuals who have lived with diabetes for many decades will often be surprised by unexpected blood glucose fluctuations. Figure 5 illustrates the two states of mind needed to deal with the vagaries of blood glucose levels.

BUMPS IN THE JOURNEY: INTENSIVE THERAPY AND HYPOGLYCEMIA

When there is more insulin in the circulation than the body needs, there is a risk that glucose levels will drop too low. The end result is a low blood glucose reaction, or hypoglycemia. Judging how much insulin to take is not always a simple task, and low blood glucose reactions are an

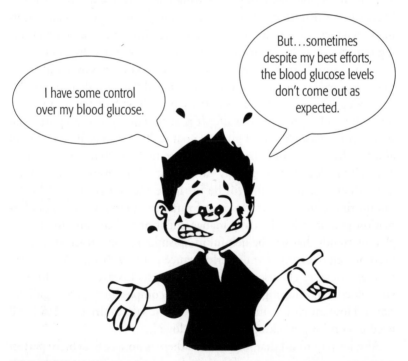

FIGURE 5 The two states of mind when dealing with the unpredictable nature of blood glucose levels.

inevitable side effect of the use of insulin to treat diabetes. The risk for hypoglycemia is increased further when you strive to keep your average glucose level close to the normal range. The common symptoms of hypoglycemia include perspiration, jitteriness, and rapid heartbeat. Sometimes if glucose levels get low enough, brain function can be impaired, disrupting the individual's ability to safely perform common activities, such as driving a car. One dangerous side effect is the inability to detect hypoglycemia, a condition known as *hypoglycemia unawareness*. With this condition, the individual is not aware when he or she is having a low blood glucose reaction. The consequence is that the glucose level can go dangerously low before it is recognized and treated.

The more common causes of hypoglycemia include the following:

- Too much mealtime insulin relative to the amount of carbohydrate eaten
- Exercise without sufficient snacking or sufficient reduction in the insulin dose
- Consuming alcohol
- Erratic absorption of insulin (this is particularly a problem with the long-acting insulin NPH and is often the underlying cause for reactions that occur overnight)
- Taking excessive amounts of insulin to bring down elevated glucose levels
- Slow emptying of the stomach

Hypoglycemia can be scary for you and for the people around you. There are a number of strategies you can use to reduce your risk of hypoglycemia. We list a few of them below. However, if you experience frequent episodes of hypoglycemia, please discuss this with your diabetes team during your next visit. They may have some great suggestions for you.

Steps to reduce the toll of hypoglycemia on you and on the people in your life:

- Connect with a diabetes self-management education program to get a better understanding about how insulin acts in the body and how to match insulin, food, and exercise. Getting involved in such an education program is often the key for many individuals with hypoglycemia. However, even with a good mastery of all of these factors, avoiding hypoglycemia can be frustratingly difficult.

- Wear a Medic-Alert chain or bracelet so that if you are ever unable to ask for help, the individuals who might come to help you (e.g., paramedics) will know that you have diabetes and will be able to care for you appropriately.
- Try to run your blood glucose levels a bit higher than usual for 24 hours after a hypoglycemic episode. This will reduce the risk of a second, more severe hypoglycemic reaction.
- Change to an insulin program that gives more predictable insulin absorption such as the pump or basal/bolus injection therapy with Lantus or Levemir. There is evidence that frequent hypoglycemia leads to hypoglycemic unawareness and that by minimizing the frequency of your hypoglycemic reactions, you can get these low blood glucose warning symptoms back. For more details on how a pump can help in this regard, see *Smart Pumping for People with Diabetes: A Practical Approach to Mastering the Insulin Pump* (Wolpert 2002).
- Use a real-time continuous glucose monitor.
- Ensure that your friends and significant others know about the treatment of hypoglycemia, including use of glucagon.
- Carry some form of fast-acting glucose with you at all times. Carrying money to buy something from a vending machine may not work if the machine is broken.
- Help your family and friends understand that you do not have 100% control over low blood glucose episodes. If they think it is entirely under your control, their worry and concern for your health and safety might be expressed as "blame and shame" (e.g. "Why do you keep doing this to yourself? Don't you care about yourself? Don't you know how ridiculous you act when you're low? Do you want to keep embarrassing me?"). It is also critical that a spouse or roommate who feels very frightened of your hypoglycemia has the opportunity to discuss this with your health care providers. This can help to prevent blood glucose levels or hypoglycemia from becoming a source of tension in your relationships with others.

WILL REAL-TIME CONTINUOUS GLUCOSE MONITORING HELP ME?

We have come a long way in the development of new technologies to help people manage diabetes. It was only in the 1970s that fingerstick blood glucose monitoring was introduced. In the past few years, real-time continuous glucose monitoring (CGM) devices have received approval from the Food and Drug Administration (FDA), and this new technology is beginning to be used by some people with diabetes.

CGM devices consist of three components: *1*) a sensor, which is a thin probe that is inserted beneath the skin (like a pump infusion set); *2*) a transmitter, which sits on top of the skin and is attached to the sensor; and *3*) a receiver, which displays new glucose readings to the user every few minutes. CGM can be a helpful tool, but it's not for everyone. In this section, we will present some background information on CGM, issues to consider in deciding whether to try this new technology, and some important pointers for successful use of CGM.

What Are the Benefits of CGM?

— Continuous monitoring gives you a continuous readout of your glucose levels, so you know if your glucose is rising or falling. Fingerstick blood monitoring gives you only a snapshot picture of your glucose levels. Your reading at bedtime is 120 mg/dl. Do you need to take a snack? If your glucose is rising, you shouldn't, but if the glucose is falling and you don't have a snack, you may end up low.

— Continuous monitors have alarms for both high and low glucose levels; these monitors can help in keeping your glucose levels out of the danger zone. If you have a history of severe hypoglycemia (reactions that have required the assistance of others for treatment) or hypoglycemia unawareness (inability to recognize your glucose level is low), CGM may be worth considering. If you're concerned about how different exercises or the timing of exercise affect your blood glucose, then CGM may be worth considering. Also, if fear of hypoglycemia is holding you back on lowering your glucose levels and A1C, CGM may be of real benefit to you.

— More information about your glucose fluctuations can translate into better decisions about how to manage your diabetes. Knowing your glucose patterns after meals can identify areas for improvement in your eating or insulin dosing.

What Is the Downside of CGM?

— CGM is not a substitute for fingerstick measurements. Current CGM devices are not as accurate as the fingerstick glucose monitors that are in widespread use. CGM devices need to be calibrated using blood measurements. In addition, before you take an insulin bolus, you need to confirm the CGM reading using a fingerstick measurement.

— CGM means you will need to wear extra hardware: a sensor/transmitter that is attached to your body.

— There is a risk of skin irritation, bleeding, or infections from the sensor.

— CGM can make diabetes seem like an ever-present part of your life. Instead of being reminded of your diabetes only the few times during the day when you check your glucose or take insulin, with a continuous monitor, you'll be getting a new glucose measurement every few minutes.

— CGM can involve expense. Currently, only a limited number of insurance companies cover this new technology.

Key Considerations Before Getting Started with CGM

1) CGM is just a tool to assist you with your diabetes self-management. Using a CGM device won't automatically lead to improved glucose control, and it will not take away the need for fingerstick monitoring.

2) You need to commit time and effort to master this technology and derive full benefit. If you have a full schedule of classes and extracurricular activities, it may not be the right time to start CGM.

3) There are several practical steps to gaining success with CGM:

   a) Initially, you will need to focus on the technical aspects of using this new technology—learning how to insert the sensors and use the controls;

   b) Understanding the differences between intermittent fingerstick blood glucose measurements and continuous sensor readings (also known as "lag"), how to calibrate the device accurately, and also how to optimize use of the alarms;

   c) How to use the continuous glucose readings to improve your glucose control.

Important Pointers for Success with CGM

1) Take it slow when you start on CGM. Initially focus on just trying to understand your glucose patterns and all the different factors (such as food, insulin, and exercise) that account for the fluctuations

in the glucose levels. Remember, improvements in diabetes control don't occur overnight—it's a stepwise process that takes time. As the continuous glucose tracings reveal where the problem areas are, you will have the information needed to tighten up your control.

2) Be prepared for a bit of an emotional rollercoaster. Starting on CGM can be an emotional experience. You'll naturally feel excited when you first begin on CGM. Then as the continuous sensor starts to reveal glucose highs that aren't apparent with just fingerstick glucose checks, it's not uncommon for this initial excitement to turn into anxiety and then frustration. This is a normal phase that usually passes. Keep in mind that the glucose fluctuations revealed by the sensor are just information to help you better control the diabetes, not a judgment on your performance in managing your diabetes.

Practical ABCs of CGM

Understanding lag

— The tip of the continuous glucose sensor sits in the space between the fat cells under the skin. This space is also known as the interstitial space.

— The glucose concentration of the fluid in the interstitial space is *not* always the same as the glucose concentration in the blood. After eating, the glucose in your meals is first absorbed into the blood and then moves into the interstitial space before being taken up by cells.

— This lag—the delay while the glucose moves from the blood into the interstitial space—can take up to 30 minutes.

What are the implications of lag?

1) When your glucose increases after a meal, this will first show up in the blood and then later in the interstitial fluid. So after a meal, you check your fingerstick blood glucose and get a measurement of 200 mg/dl, while at the same time your sensor (which measures the glucose concentration in the interstitial fluid) gives you a reading that is 30 or 40 mg/dl lower.

2) A marked difference between your fingerstick monitor and sensor can also show up when your glucose is dropping. Remember, because of lag when your glucose is dropping, your sensor (which measures the interstitial glucose) could give you a normal reading even though your actual blood glucose is quite low.

3) Finding that the fingerstick blood glucose measurement is different from the sensor does *not* necessarily imply that the sensor is inaccurate. These differences could be due to lag. Try not to lose confidence in your sensor just because it gives different readings from your fingerstick meter.

Calibration is important

Give special attention to calibration: if you do not calibrate the device properly, the sensor readings will not be accurate.

1) Carefully follow the manufacturer's instructions for calibration of the sensor.
2) Before calibrating the sensor, check to be sure that your glucose is *not* changing rapidly. The sensor readings should have changed by 60 mg/dl over the previous hour and there should be no up or down arrows.
3) Do not calibrate within 3–4 hours of a meal or an insulin bolus, during exercise, or after recovering from a low.

Situations where you must check your fingerstick glucose

— Whenever the sensor reading doesn't seem right, check your fingerstick glucose.
— If your sensor indicates that the glucose is high, you *must* confirm the reading with a fingerstick measurement before you take an insulin bolus.
— If you are driving or about to get behind the wheel and the sensor reading is normal, always check to see if there is a down arrow or if the tracing indicates that the glucose level is falling. If the glucose is falling, you *must* check your blood glucose with a fingerstick.
— If you've eaten your 15 grams of carbohydrate to treat a low, and 15 minutes later your sensor indicates that you are still low, check your fingerstick blood glucose and use this measurement to decide whether you need to take in more carbohydrate. Because of lag, when the glucose increases after a low, this will first show up in the blood and then later in the interstitial fluid; so if you rely on the sensor reading (which measures glucose in the interstitial fluid), you'd mistakenly think you needed to take in more carbohydrate to treat the low.

Be careful not to overreact to the highs by taking extra insulin

The extra information from the continuous glucose sensor can be very helpful as you strive to improve your glucose control. The most common mistake people on CGM make is to overreact to the highs shown by the sensor by taking too much insulin. Hypoglycemia is often the end result. As illustrated in Figure 6, there can be a tradeoff when using CGM to minimize hypoglycemia.

If the sensor shows that your glucose is high after a meal:

1) Check to be sure that you took an insulin bolus before the meal. Forgetting to bolus before a meal is a common error.
2) Before taking another bolus, stop to consider how much insulin you have "on board" from the previous bolus. Remember, an insulin bolus can act for 5 hours or more, so if you're high 2 hours after a meal, you usually won't need a full correction dose.

Benefiting from the alarms

The alarms are an important feature of CGM and can be helpful in reducing glucose fluctuations and hypoglycemic reactions. It can take a while to set your CGM device so that the alarms go off at the right level ("threshold"). This process involves a certain amount of trial and error.

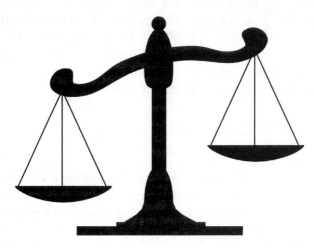

FIGURE 6 The CGM tradeoff: increased detection and prevention of hypoglycemia by the CGM alarms can be counterbalanced by an increased risk for hypoglycemia from over-bolusing.

Setting alarm thresholds involves tradeoffs

— If you set the device so that the alarm went off when your glucose rose over 160 mg/dl or dropped below 80 mg/dl, you'd be warned whenever the glucose was out of the "ideal" target range. The downside is that the alarm would go off so often that you'd probably get "alarm burnout" and end up ignoring the alarms. Avoiding alarm burnout is a key priority.

— If you set the device so that the alarm went off when your glucose rose over 250 mg/dl or dropped below 55 mg/dl, you'd have fewer alarms, making CGM less intrusive. You'll be less likely to get alarm burnout, but you wouldn't be warned of all your out-of-range numbers. In addition, because of lag, you may be significantly lower than 55 mg/dl by the time the alarm sounds.

Where to set the alarms

— **If you have hypoglycemia unawareness (inability to detect hypoglycemia) or frequent reactions that require the assistance of someone else for treatment,** you will probably want the alarm to warn you of all lows, even though you will likely get a lot of false alarms. Set the low alarm at 80 mg/dl, or even higher.

— **If you do *not* have a history of severe hypoglycemia,** it is reasonable to initially set the low alarm at 55–60 mg/dl and the high alarm at 250 mg/dl, or even higher. While you are getting used to the device, you won't be bothered by too many intrusive alarms and so there will be less chance of burnout. Later, as you use the continuous sensor to smooth out the peaks and valleys in your glucose levels, you can tighten up on the alarm settings so that they are closer to your desired target range.

MORE BUMPS IN THE JOURNEY: INTENSIVE THERAPY AND WEIGHT GAIN

As you may know, with decreasing glucose levels, there is a possibility for weight gain. However, it's important to keep in mind that there are strategies that can make it easier to control your weight through diet and exercise. But first, here is a review of how intensive insulin therapy can lead to weight gain:

- When your glucose level goes over 180 mg/dl, some excess glucose will spill over in the urine, and some of the calories taken in are lost without being used for energy. As a result, individuals with poorly controlled diabetes generally tend to eat more calories than the body needs.

■ Once glucose levels get back into target range (the goal of intensive therapy), fewer calories are lost. So unless there's less food eaten or more exercise, the extra calories may start adding up, leading to weight gain. In addition, there is evidence that when glucose levels are in the target range, calories are used more efficiently, and hence fewer calories are needed to provide energy for the body.

■ Added to this, with tight glucose control, there can be more risk for hypoglycemia (low blood glucose reactions), and eating snacks to treat these reactions means ingesting more calories (especially if you tend to eat until you feel better, instead of following the rule of taking in 15 grams of carbohydrate, waiting 15 minutes, and checking your glucose level again).

But remember that this weight gain is *not* inevitable. Changing to a basal/bolus insulin program (with either injections or the pump) can help you to keep off the weight:

■ If the Levemir/Lantus dose and pump basal rates are set correctly, there should be no need for snacks between meals, because you do not have any insulin peaking.

■ With a basal/bolus program, you can more precisely control the amount of insulin taken at mealtime, so it's easier to go on a diet. You take only enough insulin to cover what you eat. If you eat more carbohydrates, you take more insulin. If you eat less carbohydrates, you take less insulin.

■ Also, the more precise control of insulin levels with a basal/bolus program makes it easier to avoid hypoglycemia, and that means fewer snacks (and unwanted calories) to treat low blood glucose reactions.

■ Pump therapy offers an extra advantage over Levemir and Lantus when it comes to weight control. With a pump, you can reduce the basal rates during activity. This means there's less need for extra snacking to cover the activity, and so motivated individuals on the pump can use exercise more effectively to burn off unwanted calories (see Getting Physical on page 54).

Keep in mind that what you eat really counts. In the past, before basal/bolus insulin therapy and carbohydrate counting, the rule was "no sugar, no candy, no doughnuts, unless you're low!" That has now changed—carbohydrate counting offers flexibility and freedom with food choices so that you can eat whatever you want. Unfortunately, this leads a lot of individuals to suppose that "I can eat anything I want, whenever I want, in whatever amount I want, and just cover the food with extra insulin!" As you can imagine, this reasoning leads straight to weight gain.

As you move forward improving your diabetes control and mastering carbohydrate counting, try not to lose sight of the healthy eating goals all people should try to achieve—not just people with diabetes. It's easy to get so caught up in carbohydrate counting and bolus calculations, that you forget that there are also other things to be watching out for, such as fat content and calories. Fats pack in over twice as many calories as protein or carbohydrates, so restricting your fat intake can also help in keeping the lid on your overall calorie intake. Remember that alcoholic beverages can be another source of extra calories.

Perhaps during your teenage years, you, like many adolescents with diabetes, experienced increasing weight gain as your insulin dose was increased during puberty. This weight gain may have left you with an understandable fear of taking insulin. Remember that when you were going through puberty, your body was naturally less responsive (more resistant) to insulin and you required more insulin. Unfortunately, many teens do not have their insulin dose reduced after puberty, and thus, they develop the habit of "eating up" to their insulin dose. In the past, you may have felt that you had to sacrifice blood glucose control to maintain your weight.

This is why it is so important to have a nutritional consult now that you are a young adult, to ensure that your daily calorie intake is appropriate for your current insulin needs. You may feel uncomfortable discussing your weight with your health care team. Whether you are male or female, it is important for your diabetes team to understand how you feel about your weight and your shape. As a first step, speak with the nutritionist about your weight concerns. Then let all of your providers know that you want to focus on the twin goals of optimal weight *and* optimal blood glucose control. These goals are realistic when you are working in close collaboration with your multidisciplinary diabetes team.

For more pointers on healthy eating, see *The College Student's Guide to Eating Well on Campus* (Litt 2000).

SOME ADVICE FOR YOUR JOURNEY

We have just reviewed a lot of information about insulin, monitoring, and food, and it may feel like a lot to master and balance. However, instead of feeling overwhelmed, we encourage you to look at this information to change your regimen to fit your current life demands and priorities.

■ *Keep in mind that it will take a while for all your diabetes self-care tasks to become an automatic part of your daily routine.*

Achieving good diabetes control inevitably demands extra effort. Unfortunately, it's easy to get burnt out by the new demands and then, before long, decide that the effort isn't worthwhile. Don't let this happen to you. Remember that mastering the new tools of diabetes management is like learning to drive a car: initially, every action will be conscious, deliberate, and probably quite stressful. But after a while, once you've become confident in managing your diabetes, all these extra tasks will become an automatic (almost unconscious) part of your daily routine.

■ *Don't view lapses as a sign of failure.*

For most people with diabetes, the road to improvement is neither direct nor smooth. Inevitably, there will be times when other demands take a greater priority in your life than diabetes (for example, exam times or starting a new job or moving away from home). On these occasions, it's not uncommon for your focus on diabetes to lapse and for glucose control to suffer. Guard against letting these lapses lead to a total relapse, in which you lose your confidence in being able to manage blood glucose levels and begin to feel so badly about yourself that you give up, skip appointments, and avoid your diabetes team.

Where else in your life is it a failure if you do something and then decide that was not really the best choice? Aren't these situations learning experiences? Don't these experiences help us make better choices the next time? So why do we see the choices we make around diabetes care as black and white choices, when the rest of the choices we make in our lives are gray?

You may experience a "eureka" moment when you realize the importance of getting on track, but learning how to manage your diabetes does not happen overnight, or even in 6 months. For individuals making a big step, such as starting a pump or attending an instruction program on diabetes self-management, the process of mastery takes time. Keep in mind that even after that eureka moment, there are bound to be times when you lapse back into old patterns of managing your diabetes. That's normal and human. The key is to not beat yourself up for being human, but to recognize that these old patterns were not particularly useful and that the newer behaviors are more likely to help you achieve your goals.

■ *Set attainable goals.*

Mastering the intricacies of diabetes management (balancing insulin, food, and physical activity) takes time and effort. Even if your ultimate goal is an A1C of 7.0%, it's important that you start by working with your diabetes team to set an attainable goal. As you succeed in your efforts, you'll become more confident in your skills and will feel encouraged to further advance your goals. Be careful not to have unrealistic goals; aiming for something unattainable can set you up for a sense of failure and frustration, and you might reach the conclusion that the effort isn't worth it. Setting attainable goals is the key to success in all areas of life, and it doesn't make sense to see diabetes goals any differently. For example, did you begin college saying that you wanted to finish in 3 years and to make the dean's list every semester? You probably already know this is not a realistic goal. A more realistic goal when beginning college might be to strive to do your best, discover an area in which you are interested, and balance your school-work with a social life. Another unrealistic goal might be running a marathon before you've achieved the goal of running 2 miles without getting winded. A more realistic goal might be adding a quarter mile to your run each week until you've built up your stamina. Along the same lines, you do not want to begin your diabetes journey with the goals of having your A1C be under 7.0% in 6 months, or losing 10 pounds in 4 weeks. Instead, you and your team can work together at a realistic pace to lower your A1C into a safer range, or lose some weight slowly and safely. Also, remember as a practical tip that it's best to set your primary goals around new actions (or habits) rather than simply a glucose goal. Some realistic goals may be, "I will check blood sugars before I go to bed," or "I will count my breakfast carbohydrates and bolus to cover them," or "I will go to the gym with my roommate three times a week after our economics class."

■ *Everyone gets on track at a different pace.*

Some young adults reach a transition point when they begin to see getting their diabetes under control as investing in their future health. In deciding how quickly to move toward your goals, start by identifying the outside demands you must meet and the outside barriers you face (e.g., getting to work on time, meeting a deadline for class) and your own internal barriers (e.g., worrying about hypoglycemia, worrying about weight) that you will need to confront. The PAID (Problem Areas In Diabetes) questionnaire (on page 38) will help you identify some of these hurdles. Obviously, the timing has to be right, but you don't want to forever delay leaving on your journey!

Potholes and Speed Bumps Frequently Encountered on the Road of Life with Diabetes

- Worrying about the future and the possibility of serious complications
- Feeling guilty or anxious when you get off track with your diabetes management
- Feeling scared when you think about living with diabetes
- Feeling discouraged with your diabetes regimen
- Worrying about low blood glucose reactions
- Feeling constantly burned out by the constant effort to manage diabetes
- Not knowing if the mood or feelings you are experiencing are related to your blood glucose
- Coping with complications of diabetes
- Feeling constantly concerned about food
- Feeling depressed when you think about living with diabetes
- Feeling angry when you think about living with diabetes
- Feeling overwhelmed by your diabetes regimen
- Feeling alone with diabetes
- Feeling deprived about food and meals
- Not having clear and concrete goals for your diabetes care
- Having uncomfortable interactions about diabetes with family/ friends
- Not accepting diabetes
- Feeling that friends/family are not supportive of your diabetes management efforts
- Feeling unsatisfied with your diabetes physician

Items from the PAID questionnaire (Polonsky et al. 1994) are listed in order of most worrisome to least worrisome in a sample of adults with diabetes (Welch et al. 1997).

Problem Areas In Diabetes (PAID) Questionnaire

INSTRUCTIONS: Which of the following diabetes issues is currently a problem for you? Circle the number that gives the best answer for you. Please provide an answer for each question.

	Not a problem	Minor problem	Moderate problem	Somewhat serious problem	Serious problem
1. Not having clear and concrete goals for your diabetes care?	0	1	2	3	4
2. Feeling discouraged with your diabetes treatment plan?	0	1	2	3	4
3. Feeling scared when you think about living with diabetes?	0	1	2	3	4
4. Experiencing uncomfortable social situations related to your diabetes care (e.g., people telling you what to eat)?	0	1	2	3	4
5. Feeling deprived regarding food and meals?	0	1	2	3	4
6. Feeling depressed when you think about living with diabetes?	0	1	2	3	4
7. Not knowing if your mood or feelings are related to your diabetes?	0	1	2	3	4
8. Feeling overwhelmed by your diabetes?	0	1	2	3	4

	Not a problem	Minor problem	Moderate problem	Somewhat serious problem	Serious problem
9. Worrying about low blood sugar reactions?	0	1	2	3	4
10. Feeling angry when you think about living with diabetes?	0	1	2	3	4
11. Feeling constantly concerned about food and eating?	0	1	2	3	4
12. Worrying about the future and the possibility of serious complications?	0	1	2	3	4
13. Feeling guilty or anxious when you get off track with your diabetes management?	0	1	2	3	4
14. Not "accepting" your diabetes?	0	1	2	3	4
15. Feeling unsatisfied with your diabetes physician?	0	1	2	3	4
16. Feeling that diabetes is taking up too much of your mental and physical energy every day?	0	1	2	3	4
17. Feeling alone with your diabetes?	0	1	2	3	4
18. Feeling that your friends and family are not supportive of your diabetes management efforts?	0	1	2	3	4

	Not a problem	Minor problem	Moderate problem	Somewhat serious problem	Serious problem
19. Coping with complications of diabetes?	0	1	2	3	4
20. Feeling "burned out" by the constant effort needed to manage diabetes?	0	1	2	3	4

Transition Checklist: Preparing for Handling Diabetes on Your Own

Before you begin taking over your own diabetes care, ask yourself the following questions:

✓ Can I fill a prescription?
✓ Can I order my supplies before I run out?
✓ Do I have supplies to manage a low blood glucose reaction?
✓ Can I pay for or arrange to pay for prescriptions?
✓ Do I check blood glucose levels on my own or do I need reminders?
✓ Do I take my insulin on my own or do I need reminders?
✓ Do I know how to adjust my insulin based on my blood glucose reading?
✓ Do I know how to adjust my insulin based on the amount of carbohydrates I'm eating?
✓ Can I adjust my food and/or insulin based on my physical activity?
✓ Do I know when to call to make a diabetes clinic appointment?
✓ Do I know whom to call if I have an urgent diabetes question?
✓ Can I get to my diabetes clinic appointment on my own?
✓ How comfortable am I in telling my diabetes team how I have been feeling?
✓ Am I comfortable asking questions or expressing concerns about my diabetes to my diabetes team?

Preparing for the College Years

Before heading off to college, you need to pack a Campus Diabetes Kit:

- Glucose monitor and strips
- Insulin vials
- Syringes/pump supplies (reservoirs/insertion sets)
- Sharps container
- Ready source of glucose to treat hypoglycemia, such as juice, glucose tablets, and glucose gel (remember, vending machines aren't always around and aren't always reliable)
- Medic Alert identification (this may not be your first pick as a fashion statement, but if you're ever unconscious, this identification may be your lifeline)
- Important contact numbers (take a supply of business cards from your current diabetes care team to share with new health care providers and emergency room staff)
- Prescriptions for diabetes supplies

As you are getting settled into school, there are several key things that you need to do:

- Decide who and what to tell about your diabetes (see Relationships and Explaining Diabetes to Your Significant Other and Friends on page 47).
- Visit the student health service and find out how to access night, weekend, and emergency services.
- Find the cafeteria and other eating establishments, and obtain nutrition information on the foods that are served. It may be worthwhile to stock your dorm room with food.
- Prepare a Dorm Room Sick-Day Kit. This should include your sick-day guidelines for adjusting insulin, ketone strips, a thermometer, and a nutrition stock for sick days consisting of bland foods and liquids (such as juice, sugar-free beverages, crackers, and broth-based soups).

PREVENTING COMPLICATIONS

There's a good chance that you've heard more about complications from diabetes than you'd care to know.

- Yes, it's true that diabetes is the most common cause for blindness in the industrialized world.
- Yes, it's true that people with diabetes are 20 times more likely to get kidney failure than people without diabetes.
- Yes, it's true that individuals with diabetes are more likely to have limb and foot problems related to neuropathy (nerve damage) and poor circulation.

BUT, keep in mind:

- Most of the information we have about complications of diabetes is based on groups of patients who did not have access to blood glucose monitoring or intensive diabetes treatment regimens early in their course of living with diabetes.
- Complications *are not* inevitable.
- Complications *can* be prevented and sometimes reversed.
- Complications *do not* develop overnight. In fact, complications take years to develop, so occasional lapses in your diabetes control are not going to send you on the path to complications.
- *Any* improvement in diabetes control can help reduce the risk for complications.

Retinopathy (eye disease)

Retinopathy—damage to the retina, the light-sensing part of the inner eye—is one of the more common complications of diabetes. The DCCT conclusively showed that glucose control is an important factor in the development of retinopathy. For every 10% reduction in A1C, there was a 40% reduction in the risk for retinopathy. Every improvement in your glucose control counts. You don't have to achieve an A1C of 6.8% to see a benefit; just bringing your A1C from 9.5% to 8.5% will bring you a big dividend.

It should also be noted that although high glucose levels contribute to the development of eye disease, not all individuals with poorer diabetes control necessarily develop eye disease. Some 43% of the individuals in the DCCT with A1C levels over 9.5% did *not* have eye disease. In fact, only 1.8% of the patients with A1C levels over 9.5% did develop the more severe signs of retinopathy. This information tells us that it is not only higher glucose levels that lead to eye disease, but that other factors (such as high blood pressure and your genetics—what you've inherited) also play a role. Too often, individuals who get complications end up blaming themselves, and this can turn into a vicious downward spiral where blaming yourself for something you may not have been able to control can lead to feelings of depression. Often, when people feel depressed, they have less energy and less interest in caring for themselves. This can lead to spending less time and attention on taking care of your diabetes. It is important to try and prevent this cycle from developing. Keep in mind that if only some people with high A1C values develop severe retinopathy, then it makes more sense to blame your genes than it does to blame yourself and your blood glucose levels. In addition, if you do develop retinopathy, the most important thing you can do to prevent this complication from becoming worse is to continue to check blood glucose levels, continue to take your insulin, and continue to see your diabetes team.

Remember that having some eye damage from diabetes *does not* mean that you are going to become blind. With the tools available today such as laser therapy and vitrectomy surgery, the risk for marked visual loss has been substantially reduced. We'd like to mention one recent report of some 600 individuals diagnosed with type 1 diabetes between 1965 and 1984 and followed for over 20 years. Only seven individuals in this group became blind from retinopathy. Moreover, the 244 individuals diagnosed with type 1 diabetes between 1979 and 1984 had an average A1C of 8.5%, and despite this less than perfect glucose control, *none* of these individuals have developed blindness from retinopathy. All of these individuals had their blood pressure carefully monitored and had their eyes examined at least every year by an ophthalmologist (eye specialist). There is evidence that blood pressure control can have an important impact in preserving vision. In the U.K. Prospective Diabetes Study (a trial in individuals with type 2 diabetes), it was found that tight blood pressure control was associated with a 47% reduced risk for deterioration of vision.

It is important that you realize you won't notice any change in your vision when retinopathy first develops, so it's critical that you get your eyes examined at least annually. ***Early detection of retinopathy leads to early treatment, and this can preserve vision!***

How to Prevent Visual Loss from Diabetes
- If you have had type 1 diabetes for >3 years, have a dilated eye examination at least annually.
- If you do have retinopathy, check with your health care provider that your blood pressure is well controlled.
- Strive for the best glucose control you can achieve.

Nephropathy (kidney disease)

Nephropathy—kidney damage from diabetes—is one of the most feared of all potential complications from diabetes. Keep in mind that nephropathy takes years and years to develop, so kidney failure is not something that springs up suddenly without advanced warning (even though Hollywood would have you think differently!). During the earliest phase of nephropathy, the damaged kidneys start leaking small amounts of a protein called "albumin" into the urine. This is referred to as microalbuminuria, and at this early stage, the kidneys are still functioning completely normally. Although microalbuminuria is an early sign of change in the kidneys, microalbuminuria does not necessarily lead to kidney failure. Several studies have shown that individuals with microalbuminuria who take a drug known as an angiotensin-converting enzyme (ACE) inhibitor can block the diabetes from causing further damage and prevent any deterioration in kidney function. In fact, recent studies indicate that with treatment, microalbuminuria can end up disappearing. Use of ACE inhibitors, careful control of blood pressure (yes, there's the importance of blood pressure control again!), as well as improved glucose control (A1C <8%) are the key factors associated with this improvement.

Like retinopathy, nephropathy usually develops silently, so it's critical that you get your urine checked for microalbumin at least every year. *Early detection leads to early treatment, and this can prevent kidney failure!*

Don't jump to conclusions if your microalbumin test is positive

The urine microalbumin test can pick up the earliest signs of damage to the kidneys. This is obviously a good thing, since it means that you can begin treatment with an ACE inhibitor at an early time in your kidneys' long-term health, before there is any permanent change in the func-

How to Prevent Kidney Damage from Diabetes

- Be sure that your urine is checked for microalbumin annually.
- If microalbuminuria is confirmed on repeated testing of the urine, be sure that you start taking an ACE inhibitor drug.
- Be sure to check with your health care provider that your blood pressure is well controlled. You should aim to have a blood pressure <130/80 mmHg.
- Strive for the best glucose control you can achieve.

tioning of the kidneys. The downside is that sometimes the urine microalbumin test can be mistakenly positive. This false reading can occur with activity (just rushing into your appointment can be the cause), high glucose levels, fevers, urinary tract infections, or when women are menstruating. So if urine microalbumin levels come back elevated, *do not panic.* Instead, be sure this result is confirmed on repeat testing before you get labeled as having any early signs of nephropathy.

Foot Complications

You have probably heard the statistics about the increased risks for foot ulcers and amputations in some people with diabetes. Who has not heard a story about someone's great-aunt Bertha who had a foot amputated? What is less commonly emphasized is that most severe foot problems associated with diabetes are *preventable* and usually occur because of delays in seeking treatment. With some relatively simple measures, it is possible for you to ensure that you never become part of these statistics. The clinical examination performed by your health care provider when you attend diabetes clinic every 3 months can help you learn more about your risk for feet problems:

- If your pulses are okay and you can feel a 10-gram monofilament (this is a small flexible fiber used in the nerve examination), you are at low risk for running into foot problems. So don't let fears about this complication of diabetes hang over you.
- If you can't feel the monofilament, there is a risk you could injure yourself and not feel any pain. This could turn into a problem if damage to your skin or feet goes unnoticed and untreated. In

addition, if the pulses are reduced, indicating that blood flow to the feet is impaired, the healing of an injury is likely to be slowed.

How to Prevent Foot Problems from Diabetes

- Don't go barefoot, and inspect your feet and between your toes daily. These are good habits for everyone with diabetes, but especially if you have lost some sensation and don't feel the monofilament well.
- Make a habit of cutting your nails straight across. This helps prevent ingrown toenails.
- If you notice any foot problems (such as redness, an open sore, or a puncture wound), call your doctor immediately. *Early treatment can prevent foot problems from turning into a complication.*
- If you're a smoker, quit. Cigarette smoking is a major cause for circulatory problems in individuals who have diabetes.

In summary, the best investments you can make to avoid complications of diabetes are *1*) working with your diabetes team to improve your blood glucose control and *2*) continuing to see your diabetes team and get diabetes health care (including eye checkups) over the young adult years, so that you can take advantage of the newer treatments for the early signs of complications.

What Are the Chances My Children Will Have Diabetes?

That's a common question asked by individuals with type 1 diabetes. The data vary slightly from one study to another. Research performed at the Joslin Clinic indicates that if the father has type 1 diabetes, there's about a 5% risk that his children will develop this condition, whereas if the mother has type 1 diabetes, this risk is only about 2% (Warram et al. 1991, El-Hashimy et al. 1995). A similar pattern has been noted in studies from Scandinavia (Lorenzen et al. 1998). The risk also tends to vary depending on the age the parent was diagnosed with diabetes: If the father was diagnosed with diabetes before age 11, the risk is 9%, compared to 4% if the father developed diabetes after age 11. If the mother is diagnosed before age 11, the risk is 3%, compared to 2% if the mother developed diabetes after age 11. Interestingly, the data also show that if you're a woman with type 1 diabetes, the chance that your children will develop diabetes depends on how old you are when you get pregnant: if your age at the time of the pregnancy is over 25, the likelihood drops to <1%—almost as low as if you didn't have diabetes. So this might be a situation where there's a benefit to waiting.

RELATIONSHIPS AND EXPLAINING DIABETES TO YOUR SIGNIFICANT OTHER AND FRIENDS

In the past, you might have been comfortable allowing your parents to talk about your diabetes with schoolteachers, your family friends, and even with your health care team. Now this responsibility belongs to you. Or maybe you were just diagnosed and have no experience talking about your diabetes with others. Now, you are the one who needs to make a decision about the three vital issues in letting others know about diabetes: *1*) whom to tell, *2*) what to tell, and *3*) when to tell.

Whom to Tell?

Sometimes disclosing your diabetes, such as on insurance forms, driver's license applications, and college or employment health inventories, is a matter of being honest. There may be legal implications for not disclosing diabetes in these contexts. However, for other social situations, you need to develop a plan as to "whom to tell." In general, it is important to talk with those people with whom you spend a lot of time (such as roommates, close friends, lab partners, basketball coach, and teammates). Informing these people that you have type 1 diabetes, that you work hard to take good care of your blood glucose levels, but that you may at some time have a low blood glucose reaction in which you may seem "different," "confused," or even "out of it" is important. Let them know how to help you if you have a sudden low blood sugar reaction—where you keep your low blood sugar supplies and your meter and whom they should contact if it is an emergency. These steps provide a safety net for you so you can go about the business of being an active young adult.

What to Tell?

You will need to have a plan in place about what you should tell other people about diabetes. You may wish to tell others more about diabetes and that at some time you may have a low blood glucose episode and need their assistance. One guideline that may be helpful is to ask people if they have ever known anyone with type 1 diabetes, or if they have been exposed to information on diabetes? This gives you the chance to hear their beliefs and their information, as well as their misinformation, about diabetes. Then you can respond to their experience and add in the bits of information you feel are important, for example, that you wear an insulin pump to provide continuous insulin to the body, more like your friend's pancreas does, or that you check your blood glucose often so that you can adjust your management plan to avoid high and low blood glucose levels, or that there is no such thing as "forbidden" foods, and that you adjust your insulin doses based on the foods you eat.

When to Tell?

Again, it is your decision when to tell someone about your diabetes. There is of course a spectrum of times when you may want to bring up your diabetes, just as there are different times when you may wish to bring up some other personal information. For example, if your parents are divorced, you probably do not talk about this in your first conversation with someone. Rather it is much more likely that in your first conversation you tell them that you want to be a veterinarian or that you play on the basketball team. However, as a rule of thumb, if you find you are spending lots of energy keeping your diabetes a secret and feel lots of tension hiding your diabetes tasks in social situations or within a relationship, then it may be time to talk openly about your diabetes. You will develop your own timing style as your social circle expands to include new acquaintances, friends, and coworkers. Your confidence will grow as you receive responses that let you know you made the right decision.

CHANGING TIES WITH YOUR FAMILY

All of your family ties change as you move through the young adult period. Your relationships change with sisters, brothers, favorite aunts and uncles, your grandparents, and, most especially, with your parents.

It is important that as you learn how to "be more on your own," you continue to have appropriate support from your family. We have learned some lessons from young adults and their families that may be helpful for your specific family situation:

— Think about whether you are ready to meet a new diabetes care provider while you're away at school, or if you would rather keep working with your pediatric provider until you have graduated. Discuss these options with your parents and with your current diabetes team. They may each have helpful ideas and suggestions so you can make the best decision for you.

— If you choose to change to a new health care professional, keep your parents informed about your new diabetes care provider. Keep them informed about your overall health—this will help them worry less and may help to keep them off your back. When you let your parents know that you are working with a nutritionist, they can see that you are really trying to take care of yourself.

— Diabetes management and care may be expensive. Learn to talk realistically about the financial help you feel you need to take the best care of your diabetes. For example, do you have insurance coverage from your parents? Do you have health insurance through your college campus?

— Talk with your parents and siblings about all aspects of your new life, and include diabetes as you speak about your roommate, your fraternity, your class and work schedule, etc. This lets your family know that you are integrating diabetes into your new life.

— If necessary, you can keep your parents up to date on advances in diabetes treatment and research by referring them to articles, websites, and other sources of diabetes information. This indicates that you are continuing to learn about diabetes.

— If you are living at home, negotiate for the level of privacy that you need. And ask for the support you need as well.

LEARNING HOW TO BE AN EFFECTIVE PATIENT

Little attention is usually given to what it takes to be an effective patient. Graduating to a new health care provider is more than just going to see a new doctor and leaving your parents behind. You may have strong attachments to your pediatrician that have built up over many years, and you may find that "adult" doctors can be much more matter-of-fact. Keep in mind that when it comes to diabetes, the kinds of relationships individuals have with their health care providers are quite different than with other conditions. If you've broken your leg, it's your doctor who makes most of the decisions (in consultation with you) about what needs to be done to set the bones right. In contrast, when it comes to managing your diabetes, it's you who makes the day-to-day decisions, and your health care provider should be more like a coach. So you need a provider who understands that his or her role is to *guide* you in your decisions, rather than *tell* you what to do. As you move forward, it is you who will have to take charge in managing your diabetes.

It can be helpful for you to get in the habit of preparing a checklist for your visits to your health care provider:

— *Practical matters.* These matters include things such as prescriptions you need, advice about that new glucose monitor you read about, or the "travel letter" you'll need for your upcoming vacation.

— *Diabetes matters.* What has been on your mind about your diabetes, or what issues have come up since your last visit to your provider? Maybe you've decided you want to tighten up on your diabetes control and you want to discuss where to begin (if you go to the gym regularly, you may find that improving your glucose levels around exercise will help your performance, so this might be a good place to start monitoring more frequently [see page 54]; or if your supper varies a lot from day to day, you may want to learn how to adjust your insulin doses to adjust for your food intake, and seeing the nutritionist to learn about carbohydrate counting is a good place to start). Or, maybe you have concerns about how low blood glucose reactions could be affecting your relationship with your significant other; ask him or her to accompany you to your next visit. Or, maybe you have concerns about your weight (see page 32) and you want to discuss the options for dealing with this matter.

— *Prevention.* As pointed out on page 42, the complications of diabetes can be prevented and reversed. The key is early detection. Please be sure that you have a dilated eye exam and urine test for microalbumin at least every year.

Health Insurance Issues

Hopefully, in the future, everyone in this country will have comprehensive health coverage and this section will be redundant. The complexities of health insurance can be even more of a challenge during the young adult years:

- Some managed care plans won't cover nonemergency expenses out of the plan's geographic area, and if you're thinking of attending an out-of-state school or living far from home, it's important to check up on this.
- Some college-sponsored health plans do not cover preexisting conditions (such as diabetes) or the cost of outpatient prescription drugs (including blood glucose monitoring supplies). So, before enrolling in such a program, it's important to check on this.
- Many plans will allow young adults to remain on their parents' health insurance policy up until the age of 25 years, provided they are enrolled in school and remain unmarried.

Useful websites:

- For choosing health insurance: http://www.slba.com
- To learn about standards for student health insurance and benefits: http://www.acha.org/info_resources/stu_health_ins.pdf

PREGNANCY

With the remarkable technological advances of the past few decades, having a healthy pregnancy and newborn is thankfully within reach for most young women with diabetes. Success depends on having the lowest A1C level possible without undue hypoglycemia during conception. Therefore, if you choose to be sexually active, it's important to use effective contraception at all times unless you're actively trying to conceive and are in good metabolic control. Keep in mind that there are no contraceptive methods that are specifically off-limits to women with diabetes. The failure of contraception can sometimes lead to serious complications for the child of the woman with diabetes; therefore, when it comes to selecting contraception, it is important that you select methods that are known to be highly effective.

SMOKING

Cigarette smoking becomes a temptation and part of the lives of too many adolescents and young adults with diabetes, but we're not going to give you a sermon on the perils of smoking, just the sobering facts. Smoking accounts for over 400,000 deaths in the U.S. per year and is the leading avoidable cause of death in this country. In individuals with diabetes, the added risks of smoking are even greater. The risk for developing nephropathy (kidney disease) from diabetes is increased severalfold if you are a smoker. Smoking also adds to the risk of coronary artery disease, the major cause of death in people with diabetes. Smoking is a key cause for vascular (circulation) and foot problems in people with diabetes. It usually takes more than a few years for irreversible damage to set in from smoking, so it's never too late to quit smoking.

ALCOHOL

Alcohol may be part of the social scene you encounter, so it's important to understand how it can affect you and your diabetes. Binge drinking is not just something to shrug off as a passing phase in your life. The consequences—hangovers, blackouts, losing control, and giving in to unplanned and unprotected sex—can be serious. There is also evidence that excessive drinking can harm brain function. Drinking and diabetes together can be an even more dangerous, and sometimes lethal, combination.

The impaired judgment that comes from even slight alcohol intoxication can cause you to make the wrong decisions about managing your diabetes. In addition, alcohol can directly affect glucose metabolism in your body. Alcohol can have two distinctly different effects on your blood glucose levels, leading to both low blood glucose (hypoglycemia) and high blood glucose (hyperglycemia):

— **Alcohol can block the liver from releasing glucose, leading to hypoglycemia.** Earlier in this section, we mentioned that in between meals and overnight, the liver is continuously releasing glucose into your circulation. In addition to releasing glucose, your liver is also responsible for processing the alcohol out of your body. When alcohol is being metabolized by the liver (which can happen for hours after a drink), your liver is not able to produce glucose. It cannot do both jobs at once. The end result of this is hypoglycemia. Therefore, whenever you have alcohol, be prepared to snack and cut back on your insulin dose. Even one drink can impair glucose production by your liver, and this can last for hours. In addition, alcohol will block your liver from responding to glucagon, so if you go low from drinking alcohol, the glucagon emergency kit won't be much help.

— **Some alcoholic drinks contain a lot of carbohydrates, and this can lead to hyperglycemia.** Alcoholic beverages mixed with fruit juices or regular soda, beers, and sweet wines can be full of carbohydrates. The end result is an initial increase in your blood glucose level, followed by a fall in the glucose once the alcohol effect on the liver has kicked in. Avoiding hypoglycemia is the priority: when you have carbohydrate-rich alcoholic drinks, *do not* take insulin to cover the carbohydrates unless you have learned from experience that these drinks will end up increasing your glucose levels.

Some practical tips:

— Check with your health care provider for specific guidelines on adjusting your insulin and snacking for those social occasions when you are going to have a drink.

— Always have food in your stomach when you're drinking alcohol. In addition to helping to prevent hypoglycemia, food will slow down the absorption of alcohol into the bloodstream and reduce the load that reaches the liver.

— Never drink alone. Let your friends know you have diabetes, and ask them to assume that if you are acting "funny" or if you pass out, that you are having a low blood sugar reaction, not that you are drunk. Be sure that they know exactly what to do to treat a low blood glucose level and how to get you the help you need.

— Be prepared for hypoglycemia not only while you're drinking, but also for hours afterward. Be sure to have carbohydrate snacks around when you're drinking. It is often prudent to eat a large snack just before going to sleep after you have been drinking. Monitor, monitor, monitor. When going to sleep, set your alarm to wake you up a few hours later, or ask your roommate or partner to check up on you.

— Think twice before you take more than one drink. Alcohol and diabetes add up to more than double danger: intoxication leads to mental impairment, and when your judgment is clouded, you may not realize that you are going low. Others may also confuse hypoglycemia and intoxication: they may think your out-of-character behavior is due to alcohol, not realizing that you are also low and are in real need of carbohydrates.

Getting Physical

Young adulthood is a life stage when many individuals with diabetes think about introducing exercise into their daily routine. Physical activity is important for your general health and diabetes control. In addition, exercise can be a helpful way to burn off unwanted calories and to achieve your weight goals. If you are someone who exercises regularly and wants to improve your physical performance and endurance, remember that attentiveness to your glucose control is a key element to achieving this goal. A full review of all the issues relating to exercise and diabetes is beyond the scope of this book. Here, we will outline some important considerations for getting started. Please ask your health care professional for more specific guidance.

GETTING PREPARED

Preparing for physical activity is important. Most young people can safely participate in a variety of activities. Remember, though, that there are some issues to consider:
- Blood glucose monitoring is key to getting the most out of exercise and to ensuring that you exercise safely. Make a point of checking before and after the session. Sometimes it can be valuable to check in the middle. Also, if you find that your glucose tends to drop after exercise, it is important to routinely check several hours after you finish the session. Remember that exercise not only can cause you to go low, but also reduces your body's ability to recognize when your blood glucose is dropping. If you have hypoglycemia unawareness and generally only recognize when your glucose is down in the 50s or less, it is especially important that you be attentive to checking your levels before, during, and after exercise.

- Exercise can have a paradoxical effect if your diabetes is out of control. If the glucose level is very high, exercise can lead to a further increase in blood glucose and can also cause you to spill large quantities of ketones in your urine (see the American Diabetes Association guidelines on page 57 about how to determine whether it is safe to exercise when your glucose is high).
- Individuals with proliferative retinopathy (a more advanced stage of eye disease) and peripheral neuropathy (nerve damage) with reduced sensation in the feet should take certain precautions. Strenuous physical activity that involves pounding or jarring movements should be avoided. If there is more advanced eye disease, weight training (which can lead to a marked increase in blood pressure) should be limited. Low-impact aerobics, swimming, and stationary cycling are alternative activities that can provide a safe workout.

MANAGING TYPE 1 DIABETES AROUND EXERCISE

Glucose metabolism during exercise

A brief review of how glucose metabolism changes during exercise will give you the background to make the right decisions to control the diabetes when you are physically active. At the onset of exercise, muscle stores of glucose (glycogen) are the major source of fuel for the exercising muscle. Within minutes, the muscle will start covering its energy needs by taking up glucose from the bloodstream. To prevent the glucose level in the blood from dropping, the liver—which is the body's glucose reservoir—starts pouring glucose into the bloodstream. This release of glucose by the liver is triggered by hormonal changes: the key ones being the release of adrenalin (also known as epinephrine) and a drop in blood insulin levels. In people without diabetes, the pancreas shuts down soon after the onset of exercise and, within minutes, insulin levels start falling. The challenge for people with type 1 diabetes is that it's impossible for them to get their insulin levels to drop so rapidly; even after shutting off an insulin pump, it usually takes 30–60 minutes before blood insulin levels decline significantly.

Regulating glucose levels during exercise

- If your glucose level is <100–120 mg/dl when starting an activity, it is important to take in some fast-absorbed carbohydrates, such as glucose tablets; 10–20 grams is a common starting amount unless the exercise is extremely strenuous. Without this initial carbohydrate, you would be at risk for hypoglycemia because of the rapid uptake of glucose from the blood that occurs at the onset of exercise. Remember, more complex carbohydrates, such as nutrition bars, can take a while to get absorbed and generally aren't effective in preventing this initial drop in glucose levels. It can take a certain amount of trial-and-error to determine how much carbohydrate you might need to control the glucose level during more prolonged, ongoing exercise. A typical starting point is often 1 gram carbohydrate per kilogram body weight per hour of exercise.

- Reducing your insulin levels around exercise can help cut back on the quantity of carbohydrate needed to support the exercise. This can be important if you would like to use exercise to burn off calories. If you want to use this strategy and are on injections, plan your exercise sessions within 3–4 hours after your meals. This way you can cut back on your premeal fast-acting insulin bolus, allowing you to cover the fuel needs for your exercise with the meal rather than with extra snacks. Typically, the dose may need to be reduced by 25–75%, depending on the duration and intensity of the exercise. Consult with your health care professional for specific advice. If you are on an insulin pump, you can exercise between meals and cut back on the need for snacks by reducing your insulin levels with a temporary basal dose or by suspending the pump. Usually the basal rate needs to be reduced by 20–50%, starting 1–2 hours before the exercise. Sometimes, depending on the activity, you may want to remove or suspend the pump. Remember, if you are off the pump for more than 60 minutes, it is important that you check your glucose to determine if you need supplemental insulin.

- You may find that paradoxically some exercises will increase your blood glucose levels. Exercises such as sprinting or lifting weights will lead to marked release of adrenalin and this in turn triggers the liver to start producing large quantities of glucose. If the liver pours out more glucose into the blood than the exercising muscle takes up, the end result will be an increase in the blood glucose. The adrenalin surges that accompany competitive sports (and also stress) can lead to dramatic spikes in the glucose level. If your exercise routine includes both weight training and aerobics (such as fast walking or running), try doing the weights first; this way you can use the weight training to push up your glucose before you start the aerobic exercise and can reduce the quantity of snacks needed to prevent exercise lows.

- Hypoglycemia can occur long after the end of your session, so it's important to get in the routine of checking your glucose several hours after the end of exercise. After the exercise, the muscles need to replenish the glucose stores used up during the activity, and while the muscles are taking up glucose, the blood glucose levels will fall. If you exercise in the afternoon or evening, you may need to cut back on your overnight basal insulin or take a bedtime snack to prevent hypoglycemia.

AMERICAN DIABETES ASSOCIATION GUIDELINES REGARDING HYPERGLYCEMIA AND EXERCISE

- If your glucose before exercise is >250 mg/dl, check for ketones in the urine or blood. If ketones are present, *do not* exercise. If there are no ketones, you can exercise.
- If the glucose before exercise is >300 mg/dl and you do not have ketones, you should exercise with caution and check glucose levels during the exercise.

WEB RESOURCES ABOUT DIABETES AND EXERCISE

www.acsm.org (American College of Sports Medicine)
www.diabetes-exercise.org (Diabetes Exercise Sports Association)
www.childrenwithdiabetes.com/sports (Children with Diabetes)

Driving and Diabetes: A Serious Matter

Driving mishaps are more common among drivers with type 1 diabetes. Hypoglycemia is an important factor contributing to this problem because your reaction time and your judgment are impaired when you are low. Remember, your glucose level doesn't need to be very low to have a significant impact on your reaction time and on your overall driving ability. Studies indicate that driving can be impaired when your glucose level is down to only 60 mg/dl. So, the fact that you can have a normal conversation when your glucose is in this range doesn't mean you are safe to drive!

The important rules about driving and diabetes:

1. Measure your blood glucose before you start up the car and at intervals during long drives.
2. Do not begin driving if your glucose is below 90 mg/dl. Using this level as the cutoff gives you the assurance that if your glucose does happen to drop while you are driving, there's less chance that your glucose level will hit the point where you're impaired and at risk for having an accident.
3. If you develop any symptoms or signs of hypoglycemia while driving, immediately bring the vehicle to a stop at the side of the road and consume fast-acting carbohydrates.
4. After your blood glucose has returned to normal after treating a low, wait for 15–20 minutes before you start up the vehicle again and resume the journey. Remember, after the glucose level in your blood comes back into the normal range, there is a delay before your brain function fully returns to normal and you are safe to drive. Do no risk a serious accident by rushing to your destination. It is always better for you to arrive at your destination later than you had planned than to not arrive at all.

If you have diabetes and drive a truck or SUV, you need to be especially careful. The chances and severity of injury are higher after accidents involving these types of vehicles, and, in some states, the penalties for causing injury to others if you have hypoglycemia and cause a motor vehicle accident can be very harsh.

Three

For Parents: Helping Your Child During the Transition to Young Adulthood

S ince the moment your child was diagnosed with diabetes, you have probably spent countless hours thinking and worrying about your child's health and well-being. Many parents struggle with helping their children balance all of the normal adolescent and emerging adult demands (peer relationships, grades, money, dating, and career) with the demands of daily diabetes care. It may seem hard to believe that you are reading a book that talks about transitioning from pediatric to adult care. However, we want to congratulate you for showing how much you want to help your child transition to adult care in a healthy and successful way.

As you begin the task of helping your child transition from pediatric to adult care, do not lose sight of all of the normal transition issues that parents of all children should discuss. Keep in mind that conversations about adult issues are usually best done at a time when no one is in a rush, and when communication can be open and nonjudgmental. This is the time to listen to your child's thoughts and feelings about leaving the familiarity of home, friends, school, and community behind. This is also the time to reinforce many concepts you've discussed with your child throughout high school. For example, what are your thoughts and advice regarding the following?

- Choosing good friends
- Being careful when going out to parties and always going to a party with a friend who will not leave you there
- Sexual activity, sexually transmitted diseases, and birth control
- Dating safety (Have you discussed the possibility of date-rape with your child? Have you learned about college campus policies regarding this very real issue on today's college campuses?)
- Smoking cigarettes
- Alcohol use and drug use

In addition, researchers studying the relationship between adolescents/ emerging adults and their parents have found that parents who are accepting of their children's autonomy, and who help their children become independent, have confidence in their own ideas, and take responsibility for their own behaviors have children who are well adjusted (Steinberg 1990, Holmbeck et al. 2002). On the other hand, parents who tend to be emotionally controlling or who have a difficult time allowing their children to have independent thoughts and feelings tend to have children who struggle more with school and with emotional well-being (Barber and Harmon 2002).

Many of the major professional organizations concerned with adolescent health care have identified parental support as an important part of the process of transition planning (American Academy of Pediatrics, American Academy of Family Practice, and American College of Physicians– American Society of Internal Medicine, 2002). Moreover, a recent web-based survey of over 1,000 young adults with diabetes between the ages of 18 and 25 from the United States and six other countries in Europe and South America (the DAWN Youth Project) revealed that parental support was the most important influence on their ability to cope with diabetes and its daily regimen demands. These young adults, from different corners of the world, with different life experiences, all said the same thing: parental support matters! (Peyrot et al. 2008)

Parents of children with diabetes have specific concerns about their children as they move from childhood into adulthood. Parents of healthy adolescents worry about their child's ability to find and maintain a job or to manage personal finances once they become adults. Parents of adolescents with diabetes have the additional worries around their child's health. They worry about their children's ability to find appropriate diabetes health care, manage diabetes treatment away from parental support and involvement, and avoid situations that put their diabetes control and their lives at risk (Hauser et al. 1990, Seiffge-Krenke 2001).

Moreover, parents of children with chronic illnesses, who are on the brink of "emerging adulthood," often feel uneasy about the drastic changes that are about to occur with respect to their role in their child's health care. When your child was seen by the pediatric team, you were most likely the person playing the role of *historian,* reporting about daily management issues and illness episodes. You were also the *case manager,* handling daily medical and treatment needs and monitoring the supplies on-hand. In the school system, you were the *educator and advocate* for your child with respect to diabetes and its management. Finally, you were the *protector* in times of illness, crises, or other times of stress (Betz and Telfair 2007). Yet, legally, older adolescents begin to assume responsibilities and roles once held by parents when they reach the "age of majority."

So, how do you help your child begin to take on more adult responsibilities, for both the typical tasks that everyone deals with and the diabetes-specific tasks as well? In this chapter, we will offer some tips to help you guide your child toward increasing independence and confidence in the ability to care for himself or herself. This section contains a series of questions that you may have about how to help you and your child prepare for this transition.

HOW DO I SUPPORT MY CHILD WITHOUT HER FEELING LIKE I'M BEING INTRUSIVE OR NAGGING?

Open and honest communication about diabetes is more important than ever during this transition period. As a parent, now is a good time to begin thinking about how you communicate with your child:

- Are there any differences in tone or emotion when you talk about diabetes-specific topics than when you talk about other topics, such as friends, school/work, or curfews? If there are differences in the kinds of communication you have about diabetes-specific topics, this is a great opportunity to talk about this observation with your child.
- Opening up the conversation by saying something like, "I've noticed that when I ask you about diabetes, I sometimes sound really

anxious or annoyed. Have you noticed that, too?" The discussion that follows may open up an easier path for effective communication and collaboration.

- Think about possible differences between how each parent talks about diabetes-specific topics. Sometimes, parents have very different styles of communication, and each style might have its positive and negative side.

It is common for parents (who love, worry about, and want the best for their children) to express their worries and desire to be helpful in a way that children do not actually hear as being helpful. Instead, it is common for parents' attempts at helping to be misperceived by their children as intrusive, nagging, or critical. Once the parents' attempts at being helpful are seen in this negative light, the young adult's interest in collaborating and communicating with their parents is reduced. Often, arguing is the result, and then everyone in the family feels frustrated. The best way to prevent this vicious cycle is to work hard to open up lines of communication and collaboration that foster teamwork.

- Open up the conversation by saying something like, "I worry about your diabetes, maybe even more than I should, and I'd really like to be helpful to you. What things can I do to help you care for your diabetes?"
- In homes with two adults, you can ask questions like, "What are some of the things that mom does that are helpful to you? What are some of the things that dad does that are helpful? What would you like each of us to do differently?"
- Ask your child to share his or her thoughts about what will be easy with respect to his or her self-care and what will be a challenge. Ask your child for ideas on how to overcome these challenges.

Finally, when your child is living away from home (in his or her first apartment or in a dorm), it is easy for parents to begin phone and e-mail conversations by first asking about diabetes (for example, "How are your blood sugars doing?" or "How'd you decide how much to bolus for those midnight pizzas?").

- It is important to first ask your child about non–diabetes-related things. Remember that your child has a whole other life outside of diabetes, with many demands and many interests. Try to focus on these other important areas first.

HOW CAN I HELP MY CHILD FIND A GOOD ADULT PROVIDER?

To find an adult provider, the best place to start is by asking your child's current provider for some recommendations. You can also contact the local ADA office in the town in which your child lives. It's a good idea to schedule an initial interview with a potential new provider and then see if your child is interested in scheduling a follow-up visit. Sometimes it will take a few visits to a few providers before finding the right person.

Here are some things you and your child will want to find out about a new provider:

- Does this provider have experience in treating young adults with type 1 diabetes?
- Does this provider work with a multidisciplinary team or have a multidisciplinary approach to diabetes care? Specifically, are there certified diabetes educators (CDEs), dietitians, and mental health professionals who are part of the group?
- Is this provider up to date on diabetes research and the new technologies?
- Does this provider accept your child's insurance? (Remember that otherwise, you, the parent, may be financially responsible for your child's health care visits.)
- What hospital does this new provider use for admitting patients? Is it an adult-only hospital?

HOW CAN I HELP MY CHILD MAKE THE MOST OUT OF EACH MEDICAL VISIT?

There are a number of things you can do to help in this area. First, help your child learn how to be his or her own *historian:*

- What can your child tell a provider about his or her history of diabetes care and illness episodes?

- What can your child tell a provider about what was helpful and not helpful when working with the diabetes team in caring for his or her own health?
- What were the challenges?

Second, help your child learn how to be his or her own *case manager:*

- Practice making appointments.
- Practice ordering insulin and supplies.
- Discuss where to keep all information in an easy-to-access place.
- Discuss sick-day supplies and where they will be kept.
- Discuss a sick-day management plan and whom to call, and when.

Third, help your child learn how to be his or her own *educator and advocate:*

- Who needs to know that he or she has diabetes?
- What information about diabetes will need to be shared?
- How will your child handle possible misinformation or biases?

The Story of Judy and Her Mother

Judy is a 25-year-old young adult who has had diabetes since she was 9 years old. She has been overweight since she was diagnosed. Both of her parents and her younger brother are also overweight. When she was 11 years old, her parents were divorced. When she was an adolescent in middle school and high school, Judy's mother was struggling to support two children and to pay the bills. Judy's mother tried to "stay out of" her daughter's diabetes management, and she never talked with Judy about diabetes or her medical visits. Judy left home for college, and after college, she moved to New York City to work in a fast-paced publishing company.

Judy's diabetes had never been well controlled, and she received minimal diabetes care during her college years. After college when she moved to New York City, she began to feel constantly tired and found it difficult to keep up with the demands of her job. Motivated by how tired she felt and how listless she was at work, Judy sought out an adult endocrinologist in New York. This endocrinologist set rigid diabetes management goals for her and pointed out the threat of devastating complications such as kidney failure and blindness. At this time, Judy's A1C level was 13%. Judy felt scared and intimidated by this new physician's message and style, and she called her mother to ask for help and advice. Judy and her mother had not talked about diabetes since Judy left home for college at age 18. However, Judy's mother now realized that her daughter needed guidance and support, so she offered to look for other diabetes resources for her daughter in New York City. Her research led her to the conclusion that Judy should return home for a visit to reconnect with the pediatric endocrinologist she saw as a child and adolescent, and ask him for a referral for an adult endocrinologist.

Judy followed her mother's advice and came home to have a medical visit with her pediatric endocrinologist. Her doctor did not know any adult endocrinologists in New York City and in turn referred Judy to an adult endocrinologist in Judy's home city instead. Judy's mother set up a medical appointment for Judy to see this adult endocrinologist, and because Judy continued to feel frightened and overwhelmed by the idea that she may have eye or kidney damage, her mother went with Judy to see this new physician. This diabetes doctor also documented that Judy was beginning to show signs of retinopathy and nephropathy, spoke calmly with her about beginning a new diabetes management plan of intensive insulin therapy, and also referred her for an eye exam. The eye exam revealed that Judy needed laser surgery in an attempt to stop, and possibly reverse, the retinopathy damage in her eyes. Judy felt frightened and overwhelmed; however, she returned to see this new adult diabetes doctor with whom she felt she could talk about her options and her future health. After another visit with this new doctor, Judy decided she should leave her job in New York and move home to live with her mother for a while, until she could find a job and apartment. She would then be able to continue under the care of this new diabetes adult endocrinologist. Judy's mother began to take an active role in Judy's diabetes management and learned about carb counting and intensive insulin therapy along with Judy. She continued to ask Judy about the level of parental involvement that felt helpful. Judy asked her mother to go with her to all of her physician appointments, and she continued to live with her mother until she could find a job with health insurance benefits.

When Judy asked her mother to speak with a provider on her new diabetes team, Judy's mother did. However, this was always done with Judy present. Judy's mother had reentered her daughter's life at age 25 to help support diabetes management and her daughter's efforts to develop a new lifestyle that was more compatible with intensive diabetes management.

HOW CAN I HELP MY CHILD STAY CONNECTED TO THE DIABETES COMMUNITY SO THAT HE CAN ACCESS INFORMATION WHEN HE NEEDS IT?

The first thing to talk about with your child is whether he or she has *ever* felt connected to a diabetes community. Does your child feel supported by the current diabetes team? Has he or she ever participated in diabetes-related activities, such as summer camp, support groups, advocacy groups, or fund-raisers? If your child has not had a positive experience with the current provider, he or she may not know that things can be better.

Connecting to a new diabetes community can be facilitated by the Internet. Becoming part of a discussion group with a reputable website such as www.childrenwithdiabetes.com or the ADA's Youth section program, which can be accessed through www.diabetes.org, may help (for resources for young adults, click "for parents & kids" and then click "for teens"). Your child can ask for help in connecting to new providers, finding support groups, finding reliable pharmacies, and locating knowledgeable therapists.

HOW DO I STAY CONNECTED WITH MY CHILD'S DIABETES CARE?

Now is a great time to talk with your child about how much involvement he or she is willing to let you have in his or her care. Some questions you might ask include:

- Are you willing to talk about blood glucose patterns on a weekly basis with me? If not, with whom would you be willing to discuss this?
- Are you willing to allow your diabetes team to talk with me? You will need to let your child know that he or she will have to sign a form that specifically gives the diabetes team permission to share medical information with you.

■ If you are hospitalized for any reason, may I have permission to speak to the medical team members? Again, you will need to have your child complete specific forms (preferably in advance) that give permission for medical professionals to speak with you about your child's condition.

Helpful Websites for Staying Connected to the Diabetes Community

http://hctransitions.ichp.ufl.edu/hct-promo: An online brochure that describes and provides access to all of the health care transition products developed by John G. Reiss and colleagues at the University of Florida

http://hctransitions.ichp.ufl.edu/pdfs/HCT_Workbook_18up.pdf: A health care transition workbook for individuals over the age of 18, developed by John G. Reiss and colleagues at the University of Florida

http://www.sickkids.ca/good2go: A program that is being run through the Hospital for Sick Kids in Toronto, Canada

http://depts.washington.edu/healthtr: A transition program for adolescents sponsored by the University of Washington in Seattle

http://www.bcchildrens.ca/Services/SpecializedPediatrics/YouthHealth: A site developed by the Youth Health program site at British Columbia Children's Hospital

http://jaxhats.ufl.edu: The website from a clinic developed by the Jacksonville Health and Transition Services (JaxHATS)

http://www diabetes.org: The website of the American Diabetes Association, containing communities for parents, teens, and young adults as well as excellent sections on advocacy and employment discrimination

http://www.childrenwithdiabetes.com: A website that offers education and support to families living with type 1 diabetes, also offering scholarship information for youths with type 1 diabetes and yearly conferences in different places around the United States for families with type 1 diabetes

WHAT CAN I DO TO HELP MY CHILD PLAN AHEAD FOR COLLEGE?

It may be helpful to have a discussion about the many choices that are ahead for your child. Some diabetes-specific questions you might like to discuss as a family include:

- Whom do you tell that you have diabetes?
  - Your roommate?
  - Your R.A. (residence hall advisor)?
  - New friends?
  - Professors?
  - Health services on campus?
- Do you want to have a letter from your diabetes team that states that you have diabetes, so that you can give it to professors or other adults that might be responsible for you?
- Are you comfortable carrying carbs with you while you're running around campus?
- How will you treat lows?
- Will you have time to eat in between classes?
- Do you need a refrigerator in your dorm room to store supplies/ keep food?
- Where will you store your syringes so that no one else can use them?
- Where will you keep your sharps box?

HOW DO I COPE WITH MY CHILD'S BURGEONING INDEPENDENCE?

You have been preparing your child for independence for many years. This is a process where you are teaching your child how to be thoughtful when he or she makes decisions, how to plan ahead for potential struggles, and how to become a great problem-solver. As children grow up, parents begin to let them handle their own difficulties and challenges. You have helped your child learn how to effectively manage the natural ups and downs of life. You are no longer "fixing" things for them, but encouraging them to figure out their own solutions. However, many parents find that when their child moves away from home, the parent's level of stress increases. Sometimes this is a result of the huge technological changes in our society. With cell phones, texting, e-mails, and instant messaging, we now have immediate access to our children, and they have immediate access to us. So, if your child is distressed about an argument with a roommate, or about a grade on an exam, they are contacting you at the very moment they are the most upset. Parents find that being far away from their child, yet hearing the intensity of their distress, is extremely upsetting. Often, parents will say that they remain upset for days over these phone calls or messages, while their children have moved on within hours. We encourage parents to talk with their children about this situation and discuss issues of when to call/contact you. Sometimes, encouraging your child to wait just a few hours to think the difficulty through before contacting you not only can save you some emotional upheaval, but also can encourage your child to use his or her own problem-solving skills.

Especially with respect to solving diabetes-related problems when away at college, you need to help your child to develop other resources for support and problem-solving. Working through the college infirmary, can your child locate another student on campus who is living with diabetes? Another option is for your child to reach out to the familiar pediatric team of providers your child trusts. (However, this option needs to be discussed in advance with your child's diabetes team to make sure they are open to receiving calls from your child.) As a last resort, you can ask your pediatric team to identify a diabetes resource in the new community whom your child can contact for problem-solving.

Four

Clinical Principles for the Health Care Professional

IMPLICATIONS IN CARING FOR YOUNG ADULTS WITH DIABETES

This section is intended for health care professionals who take care of young adults with diabetes. Below, we provide background on the important issues that will often need to be addressed in the care of the young adult with diabetes, and we outline guiding principles to assist in the care of these patients.

Young adults with diabetes are a high-risk group. As highlighted by the follow-up data from the DCCT, the demands and challenges of the young-adult phase of life can detract from a focused commitment to diabetes care. Four years after completion of the DCCT, the cohort who had entered the trial as adolescents were young adults (mean age of 26 years) with a mean A1C of 8.4%, similar in both the conventional and intensive groups (Diabetes Control and Complications Trial/ Epidemiology of Diabetes Interventions and Complications Research Group 2001). In contrast, at this stage after completion of the trial, the adult cohort now with a mean age of 38 years had mean A1C values around 8.0% (Diabetes Control and Complications Trial/Epidemiology of Diabetes Interventions and Complications Research Group 2001). It is noteworthy that individuals who were in the intensive treatment arm of the DCCT had poorer glycemic control as young adults than as adolescents. These findings indicate that intensive care of adolescents with diabetes does not necessarily set the stage for optimal glucose control during young adulthood and underscore the need for focused intervention to help young adults successfully cope with the transition to independent self-care.

Young adults with diabetes face an increased risk for premature morbidity and mortality. The British Diabetic Association Cohort Study found that in the 20- to 29-year-old age-group, mortality is increased threefold in men and sixfold in women compared with the general population (Laing et al. 1999a). Acute complications were the major cause for mortality in this age-group, with 68% of diabetes-related deaths being certified as due to hypoglycemia and ketoacidosis (Laing et al. 1999b). Further study of this cohort has identified that several psychosocial factors—including living alone, past drug abuse, and a history of psychiatric referral—are significant contributors to this increased mortality from acute diabetes-related events (Laing et al. 2005). Population-based studies from Scandinavia also indicate that acute metabolic complications are the most common cause of death in the age-group under 30 years of age and also show an association with alcohol/drug misuse and mental illness (Dahlquist and Källen 2005, Waernbaum et al. 2006, Wibell et al. 2001). From 30 years of age onward, cardiovascular disease is the predominant cause of death in individuals with type 1 diabetes (Skrivarhaug et al. 2006). Risk for accelerated macrovascular disease underscores the importance of early treatment of dyslipidemia in young adults with diabetes (Wadwa et al. 2005).

The microvascular complications of diabetes may present during the young adult period. Follow-up data from the nationwide Diabetes Incidence Study in Sweden, which registers all new diabetes diagnoses in the 15- to 34-year-old age-group, indicates that 6% of the cohort diagnosed with type 1 diabetes in 1987–1988 had incipient or overt nephropathy (i.e., micro- or macroalbuminuria) 10 years later. Over half of the cases of renal disease occurred in individuals in the highest quartile of A1C values (>8.2%) (Svensson et al. 2003). The same follow-up study reported that 5% had moderate nonproliferative retinopathy and 2% had proliferative retinopathy 10 years after diagnoss (Henricsson et al. 2003). Other studies involving young adult populations have shown a higher prevalence of eye disease. Maguire et al. (2007) reported that in an Australian young adult cohort with type 1 diabetes, 15% had a history of moderate retinopathy and 10% had a history of severe retinopathy requiring laser. A U.K. study of young adults with type 1 diabetes in poor glycemic control found that 34% had background retinopathy, 8% had preproliferative retinopathy, and 25% had undergone laser therapy (Bryden et al. 2003). Young adults who developed complications had significantly worse mean A1C levels during the 11-year period preceding the evaluation (9.9% versus 8.0%). As mentioned in Part 1, the studies of Bryden et al. (2001) indicate that behavioral problems during adolescence are a predictor of poorer glycemic control in young adulthood and a significant predictor of serious microvascular complications (Bryden et al. 2003). Weight gain during the transition from adolescence to young adulthood can be an important factor contributing to poor ongoing diabetes self-management and adherence and may set the stage for insulin restriction in an attempt to lose weight. Over one-third of a sample of adolescent and young adult females with type 1 diabetes in the United Kingdom acknowledged intentional reduction or omission of insulin to control weight (Peveler et al. 2005). Similarly, a study at the Joslin Diabetes Center in Boston documented that about 30% of women with diabetes, between 13 and 60 years of age, who were surveyed reported that they withheld insulin to lose weight (Polonsky et al. 1994). As mentioned in Part 1, an 11-year follow-up assessment of this cohort revealed that those women who restricted insulin for weight control had significantly more diabetes-related complications and a threefold greater risk of death than the women who did not restrict insulin (Goebel-Fabbri et al. 2008).

DEPRESSION IN THE YOUNG ADULT WITH DIABETES

Depression rates in people with diabetes are 1.5–2 times higher than in the general population (Lustman et al. 2002). Therefore, it is important for the clinician who cares for young adults with diabetes to be alert to the symptoms that could be indicative of depression. Certain symptoms of clinical depression, such as lethargy, fatigue, and loss of interest in typical activities, mimic the symptoms of chronic hyperglycemia, so it is sometimes difficult to diagnose depression in a young adult in poor metabolic control. It has been reported that adolescents with diabetes who are depressed frequently suffer depression during the young adult years (Wysocki et al. 1992). Because depression is a strong barrier to successful diabetes self-care, it is important for the diabetes clinician to have a relationship with a mental health provider (social worker, psychologist, or psychiatrist) who is knowledgeable about diabetes and depression so that referrals can be made in a timely way when the clinician suspects major depression during the vulnerable period of young adulthood.

Depression Is a Continuum of Symptoms

- Occasional, short-lived periods of feeling down, irritable, stressed, or out-of-sorts; short-lived feelings and inconsequential feelings; or a bad day followed by a good one is not clinical depression, but rather a transitory state.
- Major depressive disorder (MDD) is a serious, sometimes life-threatening cluster of mental and physical symptoms. It is important for clinicians to be aware of the symptoms of MDD.

The five diagnostic criteria for MDD according to the DSM-IV-TR (*Diagnostic and Statistical Manual of Mental Disorders,* 4th ed., Text Revision) (American Psychiatric Association 2000) are as follows:

1. **One** of the following:
   Depressed mood
   Markedly diminished interest or pleasure in most activities
2. **Four** of the following:
   Significant weight loss or gain
   Insomnia or hypersomnia
   Psychomotor agitation or retardation
   Fatigue, loss of energy
   Feelings of worthlessness or guilt
   Impaired concentration or indecisiveness
   Recurrent thoughts of death or suicide
3. Symptoms must be present most of the day.
4. Symptoms must be present nearly daily for 2 weeks or more.
5. Symptoms must result in significant distress or impairment and not be due to medications, medical conditions (for example, chronic poor diabetes control), or bereavement.

CATHY'S STORY: A Complex Case of Depression in a Young Adult with Type 1 Diabetes and Multiple Psychosocial Challenges Who Recently Transitioned to Adult Care

Cathy is a 24-year-old woman who was diagnosed with type 1 diabetes when she was 12 years old. She came to an adult diabetologist after 12 years of infrequent and unsatisfying diabetes medical care from a community pediatrician. Her current A1C is 12%.

Cathy presents as a very immature young woman, with some cognitive delays and with no life plans or goals. She currently lives at home with her parents. She also has a history of sexually abusing a younger brother when she was 13 years old and her brother was 10 years old.

The adult diabetologist was worried that Cathy's cognitive problems and flat affect and mood might be due to her years of chronic poor glycemic control, so he addressed this concern first. However, in working with Cathy to improve her control, it became clear to the physician that her cognitive skills were so limited that her parents would need to be involved in her diabetes treatment plan.

In a meeting with Cathy and her parents, the father presented as a very overprotective and somewhat sexually inappropriate man with respect to his interactions with his daughter. Cathy's father at first claimed that he currently supervised all of Cathy's injections. However, when the physician asked for more details and blood glucose log information, the truth was revealed—that Cathy had been responsible for all of her own injections and monitoring since she was diagnosed at age 12 years. The physician worked to involve Cathy's mother in giving insulin injections, and both parents were required to receive basic diabetes education and skills training.

After 4 months of Cathy's mother giving all injections and checking blood glucose levels, the diabetologist was able to transition Cathy to a multiple-injection regimen and her A1C improved to 8.2%. At this point, the diabetologist referred Cathy to a psychologist for an evaluation.

After meeting for several sessions with Cathy and her parents, the psychologist made a diagnosis of major depression disorder (MDD), posttraumatic stress disorder (PTSD) due to being both a victim and a perpetrator of child sexual abuse, and secondary significant cognitive delay and emotional immaturity. The psychologist recommended continued family therapy and referred Cathy to a psychiatrist for medication management.

For 6 months, Cathy took antidepressant medication and attended weekly family therapy. She also enrolled in a sheltered workshop for basic employment skills training and moved into a halfway home, where her injections could continue to be closely supervised. These actions prompted Cathy to have continued excellent glycemic control, with A1C values <8.5%. However, Cathy could not yet be in charge of diabetes management tasks. Yet with the close involvement of a supervisory staff at the halfway house, and living away from the parental home, Cathy continued to improve and was soon able to be employed in an assembly-line factory position.

While employed at the factory, she met and married a young man who was also employed there. Her physician asked that Cathy's fiancé come in for diabetes education and training in insulin injections and blood glucose monitoring. After she was married, Cathy's husband assisted with all insulin injections, and she continued under the care of the adult diabetologist. Cathy also continued to undergo individual therapy and take antidepressant medication supervised by a psychiatrist.

CLINICAL FOCUS DURING THE YOUNG ADULT PERIOD

Although the population groups examined in the published studies reviewed in the introductory part of this chapter may not be broadly representative of patients from elsewhere, the findings from these investigations highlight the important clinical issues and high-risk behaviors that should be addressed by the clinician taking care of the young adult with diabetes. Evaluation of the young adult should include specific attention to identifying factors (such as alcohol and drug abuse, mental illness, and insulin restriction) that lead to neglect of self-care tasks and increased mortality from acute metabolic complications in young adults with diabetes. A nonjudgmental and supportive approach by the clinician can be critical in making the young adult feel comfortable about acknowledging insulin restriction. College students with diabetes identify several factors that can be barriers to optimal self-care, including time constraints, erratic schedules, food choices, concerns about hypoglycemia, and absence of social support. Motivators for improved diabetes control cited by this age-group tend to be short-term issues, in particular, feeling better physically and being able to participate in normal activities with their peers (Wdowik et al. 1997). Mellinger (2003) has outlined practical issues that need to be addressed in preparing students with diabetes for life at college. Important issues that deserve special consideration include alcohol (which is a major factor contributing to hypoglycemia in the college age-group), sexual health, and having a sick-day diabetes management plan. Understanding the specific factors that detract from a focused commitment to diabetes self-care and the individual motivators for improved control are the foundation in developing a realistic treatment plan with attainable goals.

MICHAEL'S STORY: A Case of Balancing Competing Demands

Michael is a freshman at a college 300 miles from his parents' home. He has lived with diabetes for 8 years. Before he went to college, his A1C levels were running around 8.5%. Michael is enrolled in the honors program at his school and is hoping to major in chemistry. He is also on the school's swim team, and he received a scholarship to join the swim team. He is living in a dorm and has made a large group of friends from his honors program and from the swim team. He is finding it difficult to balance the rigorous academic demands with the rigorous swim team demands, as well as balance the different social schedules of his friends from these two different areas of his life. He is also very interested in a girl named Emma he met in calculus class and would like to ask her out. During the third week of the first semester, Mike suffered a significant hypoglycemic reaction in the lobby of his dorm. All he remembers is that EMS personnel were kneeling next to him and a large crowd of his peers were all around him. He is terrified of having a low blood sugar reaction again, since this event continues to be the talk of the dorm, his coach has mentioned it to him a few times, and he is embarrassed. When he came home over winter break, his A1C level was up to 11%.

Michael's parents listen to his story about the embarrassing low blood glucose reaction in front of all of his friends. They understand that he is now running his blood glucose levels higher to avoid all of the hypoglycemia that has resulted from his rigorous daily swim practices. Michael also tells his parents that his swimming is being affected by the higher blood glucose numbers he has been running. Michael's dad suggests that Michael give a call to either his physician or his diabetes educator from his pediatric diabetes team to get their help in problem-solving this dilemma. His diabetes educator, who has known the family for 8 years, schedules an appointment with Michael to help him consider all of his options. One suggestion she has is that Michael begin to use a pump, for which he can program a lower basal insulin infusion rate during and after swim practices. Michael had never worn a pump and did not like the idea of being "attached" to a machine. However, his educator emphasized that pump therapy would provide him the safest guarantee of meeting both of his goals—optimal A1C and avoidance of serious low blood glucose reactions. Because Michael was home for 2 weeks over winter break, he decided to attend the class to learn intensive management using the pump, and he even learned that he could wear his pump in the pool if he wanted to.

Over this winter break, Michael was trained on the insulin pump and began to swim at the YMCA pool in his hometown to try this treatment method out. It seemed to solve the problem of low blood glucose lags very well, and Michael could feel that his strong breast stroke was coming back. However, Michael was nervous about how his peers, and especially Emma, would react to his pump. Michael talks with his educator about these concerns and she encourages him to be proactive and explain the pump to his coach, his roommate, and his closest friends and explain to them how the pump will help to prevent the serious low blood glucose reactions that happen when he has swim practices daily. Michael feels very encouraged and ready to return to school and improve both his swimming strokes and his blood sugar levels.

IMPORTANCE OF THE BEHAVIORAL/ DEVELOPMENTAL CONTEXT

The unique needs of emerging adults with diabetes described above pose a challenge to both pediatric and adult care systems, since these individuals fall outside the focus of the neatly divided pediatric and adult tracks (Wolpert and Anderson 2001). The standards of medical care propagated by the American Diabetes Association include specific recommendations for several special population groups (including children and adolescents, preconception, and older individuals) (American Diabetes Association 2008); however, these guidelines make no mention of the special needs of young adults with diabetes and of the related importance of considering behavioral and developmental issues in the evaluation and treatment of the young adult patient. However, this tendency to neglect the post-adolescent youth is changing in the American Diabetes Association, as demonstrated by their current Youth Strategies Committee, which defined their target group as children, adolescents, and young adults with diabetes up to 30 years of age (Anderson 2008).

The conclusive evidence from several multicenter trials establishing a causal link between glycemic control and the microvascular complications of diabetes has highlighted the importance of the A1C level as a key predictor of future health. Inevitably, the focus of the interaction between the clinician and patient has increasingly become directed around blood glucose monitoring records and A1C measurements. However, despite the evidence that "metabolic control matters," tight glycemic control remains an elusive goal for many individual patients. Several studies have shown that diabetes self-management education without interventions to reinforce behavior change does not lead to sustained improvement in glycemic control and underscore the importance of considering the behavioral and developmental hurdles to maintaining tight glycemic control in the young adult patient (Peyrot et al. 2008). Vinicor (1994), in reviewing the barriers to translation efforts, emphasized that since the patient with diabetes must take responsibility for his or her own care on a daily basis, successful approaches for the implementation of diabetes management must have a major focus on strategies that promote change in self-care behavior.

The importance of a developmental and behavioral framework when helping patients transition was underscored by Dovey-Pearce et al.

(2005), who concluded their series of focus groups with young adults with diabetes by recommending that "health professionals, by becoming more developmentally aware, could help buffer young people from the overwhelming demands of the health care system while encouraging and supporting them to gain the knowledge, skills, confidence, and experience they need to become committed and active partners in the process, and more effectively engaged in their health care." This task may be easier said than done, however, since health professionals may have different expectations regarding their role as providers, depending on how and where they trained. For example, Telfair et al. (2004) assessed provider perceptions regarding transition services, and although most agreed that transition programs were necessary, few did anything to facilitate the transition process. In addition, those who care for both adolescents and adults expected to see the patient with their parent, whereas those who cared only for adults expected to see the adolescent alone. Individuals trained as pediatric providers tend to worry about the quality of adult care services available to their patients (Freed and Hudson 2006, Stabile et al. 2005, Visentin et al. 2006). This worry translates to outcomes, since it appears that when pediatric providers express skepticism regarding access to quality care, it impedes transition (Brumfield and Lansbury 2004). Pediatric providers' concerns regarding their patients' access to providers (Bjornsen 2004, Scal et al. 1999) and their concerns about their patients' access to funding and insurance coverage (LoCasale-Crouch and Johnson 2005, Scal et al. 1999) also affect their participating in transition planning. Individuals trained as adult providers also have concerns about transitioning care, including the need to have teaching materials that are specifically geared for young adults/adolescents that can be use in their clinics (McDonagh et al. 2004, Shaw et al. 2004).

CLINICAL CHALLENGES OF THE EARLIER PHASE OF YOUNG ADULTHOOD

For the adolescent with tight glycemic control, the transition to young adulthood will often have only a minimal effect on established routines of diabetes self-care. However, for the vast majority of adolescents progressing to young adulthood, their growing responsibilities will often be a distraction from the demands of managing the diabetes. And even in the face of suboptimal glycemic control, some of these young adults will not be receptive to making major changes in their diabetes regimen. Reconciling this misfit between the demands of diabetes self-management and the developmental maturity of the young adult is a major challenge for the clinician.

It is not uncommon for the young adult patient and the health care provider to have different perceptions of the important priorities in care. In contrast to the patient presenting at a time of crisis (such as the diagnosis of diabetes or the onset of complications), who usually expects the physician to be directive and present a comprehensive treatment plan, the asymptomatic young adult who is "graduating" from the pediatrician may not recognize the need for major changes in his or her diabetes regimen. Some young adults may perceive unrealistic expectations and demands by the new physician, with whom they have not yet developed a bond of confidence and trust, as an intrusion on their sense of autonomy and personal control, and this can lead to estrangement from follow-up and care.

REALISTIC EXPECTATIONS AND GOALS FOR THE CLINICIAN DURING THE EARLIER PHASE OF YOUNG ADULTHOOD

- The clinical evaluation should include an assessment of the barriers to care and the competing life demands of the young adult. The treatment approach and plans will need to be tailored according to the expectations and receptiveness to change of the young adult—Is the patient just graduating to an adult provider? Is he or she expecting change? Is he or she receptive to change? (See Uncover Barriers to Intensive Therapy on page 84. The evaluation process can be aided by having the patient complete the Problem Areas In Diabetes [PAID] questionnaire on page 38.)
- The focus in care may need to be directed at ensuring that the young adult has continued medical follow-up with annual urine microalbumin measurements and dilated eye examinations and counseling concerning issues such as sick-day diabetes management, preparing for college, coping with the impact of diabetes on relationships, how to be an effective patient, contraception, smoking, preventing alcohol-induced hypoglycemia, and the risks of binge drinking. (Part 2 presents an overview for the young adult

patient on the importance of preventive screening and the subjects that might be covered in a counseling session.)

- Establishing a strong relationship based on acceptance and mutual respect can be critical to ensure *1*) continued follow-up and *2*) influence that *over time* can be directed to promote improvements in self-care behavior. Retrospective studies have established that irregular clinic attendance and loss to medical follow-up is an important predictor for the development of diabetic nephropathy (Krolewski et al. 1985). As outlined in Part 1, with maturation, the focus of the young adult shifts toward making choices and plans for the future, and this will usually be accompanied by receptiveness to changing self-care behavior and improving glycemic control. This transition can be a rewarding window of opportunity for the clinician to shape the behavior that will determine the future health of the young patient. And the efforts invested by the clinician in developing a trusting relationship with the patient will often begin to reach fruition at this later stage.

- A fundamental role of the health professional in diabetes care is to serve as the patient's guide in making informed choices about living with diabetes. As mentioned earlier, adolescents and young adults are usually very sensitive to issues of control and personal autonomy; therefore, highlighting your recognition that responsibility and control belong to the patient can be very helpful in establishing a collaborative relationship. We have also found it helpful when a provider explicitly describes himself or herself as the patient's "coach."

As pointed out by Anderson and Funnell (2000), the traditional model of medical care in which the health care provider prescribes the treatment plan and expects patients to blindly follow this prescription does not conform to the practical realities of living with diabetes, where young adult patients must assume responsibility for their own care on a daily basis. As a counterpart to the new relationship that evolves between parent and child during the transition from adolescence to young adulthood, this phase of development should be accompanied by a reorientation of the provider-patient relationship. We recommend a collaborative model with the provider guiding (rather than directing) the patient in his or her choices about living with diabetes. An accepting and nonjudgmental approach by the clinician (i.e., being respectful of the patient's concerns and views and recognizing the extra burden and effort involved in living with diabetes) can be an important underpinning to building a strong relationship. If compliance with the provider's goals becomes the condition for approval, and lapses in self-care and glycemic control are met with belittling or threatening comments, there is a risk that this will reinforce the patient's personal sense of discouragement and lead the patient to further disengage from care and medical follow-up. (A perspective for the patient on how to prevent backsliding from turning into failure is presented under Some Advice for Your Journey on page 35).

BUILDING MOTIVATION TO CHANGE SELF-CARE BEHAVIOR

The clinician's task in building motivation and overcoming ambivalence about change in self-care behavior is complex and sometimes daunting. There are several considerations in this process.

Different Perspectives About Intensive Therapy

It is clear from clinical practice that simply telling patients about the benefits of intensive therapy is rarely effective in persuading them to change their self-care behavior. Developing effective communication between provider and patient requires a convergence of perspectives and goals. The physician's perspective, shaped by the ADA Clinical Practice Recommendations, will often focus on setting up the treatment plan, i.e., telling patients what they need to do to improve diabetes control. In general, the clinician's perspective tends to emphasize the benefits of good glycemic control while undervaluing the extra demands and personal costs. In contrast, the patient's perspective is often shaped by critically weighing the implications of a particular therapy, and he or she is often more concerned about the immediate costs, demands, and sacrifices, while tending to lose sight of possible long-term benefits.

These contrasting perspectives highlight two important considerations:

- Although improved glycemic control may be the key therapeutic endpoint, the focus in care should not be directed exclusively around blood glucose management but should also be framed in terms of *making the diabetes more manageable.*

■ In introducing the patient to the tools of intensive diabetes management, the message of the provider needs to be reoriented to the patient's perspective, i.e., the more immediate and direct benefits of multiple injections and pump therapy to provide a *flexible, individualized* treatment program that fits into the demands of life.

Focus on the more immediate benefits.

⇓

Overcome ambivalence about change.

⇓

Promote engagement in self-care.

⇓

Improvement in glycemic control.

Uncovering Barriers to Intensive Therapy

Some patients may have personal barriers that stand in the way of improved diabetes control. Helping patients to identify and overcome these hurdles can be a critical element in the path to intensifying glycemic control. Some of the more common barriers that are encountered in clinical practice include the following.

Misconceptions that equate intensive diabetes control with intensive self-control

Explain to the patient that every 1% decline in A1C is only equivalent to reducing his or her mean blood glucose level by about 30 mg/dl (Nathan et al. 2008) and is associated with a greater than 40% decline in risk for microvascular complications (Diabetes Control and Complications Trial Research Group 1995, Lachin et al. 2008). This explanation will often help the patient to appreciate that intensive glycemic control is within reach and that even modest improvements in control can have a major impact on his or her future health. (A perspective for the patient emphasizing this point is presented in Preventing Complications on page 42.)

Fear of hypoglycemia

A history of severe hypoglycemic reactions should prompt consideration of whether fear of hypoglycemia underlies reluctance of the patient to intensify therapy (Thompson et al. 1996). In many of these cases, there is a history of hypoglycemic reactions that have caused personal embarrassment to the patient or triggered interpersonal conflict, and directed questioning may be necessary to uncover this barrier. (A perspective for the patient outlining measures for managing and coping with hypoglycemia and hypoglycemic unawareness is presented on page 24.)

Unrealistic expectations leading to perfectionism

Formative experiences with diabetes professionals who have set unattainable treatment goals and expectations can leave the patient with a legacy of unrealistic perfectionist strivings that lead to frustration and disengagement.

KATE'S STORY: Pediatric Diabetes Care and the Young Adult Transition

Kate was diagnosed with diabetes when she was 9 years old, in the third grade. For 10 years, she saw a pediatric endocrinologist who insisted that Kate monitor her blood glucose four to six times per day and repeatedly warned Kate and her parents that her blood glucose levels must all be under 120 all the time to prevent diabetes complications. Although Kate had several severe insulin reactions in school, her pediatric endocrinologist did not change her blood glucose targets or her insulin dose.

Especially during her adolescent years, Kate's blood glucose values were seldom under 200. She was hospitalized four times for diabetic ketoacidosis, and she continued to gain unwanted weight. Kate's parents were frightened and frustrated and reminded her all the time about the threat of diabetes complications. Soon Kate stopped monitoring her blood glucose completely and wrote down "appropriate" numbers in her logbook to please her parents and doctor. When her A1C became higher and higher, the pediatric endocrinologist wrote letters to Kate and her parents warning her of her risk of eye and kidney disease and accusing Kate of falsifying her blood glucose readings. Her parents tried to "ground her" when she failed to monitor her blood glucose, but soon they simply gave up in the face of Kate's rebelliousness.

Kate went to a local community college, lived at home, and continued to see her pediatric diabetes provider. After receiving her 2-year degree in accounting, at age 19, Kate began to work in a demanding business and quickly excelled. Because Kate was now fully supporting herself, she felt that she was an adult, and she stopped seeing her pediatric diabetes provider. However, over the next several years, her frequent hypoglycemia and unstable blood glucose levels led to many absences from work. Kate's supervisor put her on probation and urged her to get better diabetes care. Under the threat of losing this excellent position, Kate and her parents decided she should see an adult diabetologist.

At this point in her journey with diabetes, Kate, now age 23, did not monitor her blood glucose and often reduced her insulin to control her weight. Kate was exhausted from years of failing to meet her parents' and doctor's expectations, and she was completely disengaged from her diabetes management. Kate was dissatisfied with her frequent hypoglycemia and chronic fatigue, which interfered with her social life and work performance, and she was unhappy about her weight; however, she did not connect these problems to her diabetes. She felt guilty and frightened about her years of poor diabetes self-care.

When she met with her new adult diabetologist, Kate appeared listless, bland, and unable to express any feelings about diabetes or her past diabetes care. To work through this burnout and discouragement, the new adult provider negotiated diabetes management goals that spoke to Kate's immediate concerns—weight gain, fear of hypoglycemia, and feeling chronically discouraged. Working together with her adult team, Kate learned to set small goals that allowed her to make steady progress as she worked to maintain her weight and healthy blood glucose levels.

Concerns about weight gain associated with intensification of glycemic control

Misuse of insulin can be an effective weight loss strategy, and the possibility of intentional under-dosing or omission of insulin should be considered if the patient has persistent unexplained poor glycemic control despite intensive diabetes self-management education and follow-up.

Eating Disorders in Young Adults with Diabetes

The Facts

- Although there is some controversy whether there is a greater prevalence of clinically diagnosable eating disorders (anorexia nervosa, bulimia nervosa, binge eating disorder) in individuals with diabetes, recent research has shown that young women with diabetes have 2.4 times the risk of developing an eating disorder than age-matched women without diabetes (Jones et al. 2000). Importantly, several studies have shown that about 30% of all women taking insulin struggle with "subclinical" symptoms of "disordered eating," such as restrictive eating, a preoccupation with weight and shape, feelings of guilt after eating, and strategic misuse of insulin for weight control (Polonsky et al. 1994).

- Clinically diagnosable eating disorders such as anorexia and bulimia as well as "subclinical disordered eating attitudes and behaviors" present a serious health risk to the patient with diabetes. Disordered eating is associated with poor metabolic control, problems in adherence, depression, increased risk of diabetic ketoacidosis (DKA), and increased rates of microvascular complications in women with diabetes. Misuse of insulin for the purposes of weight control is such an effective weight loss strategy, that it is almost impossible for young women to stop this high-risk behavior on their own.

- Therefore, it is critical that diabetes clinicians understand the following:

  1) How to prevent the development of disordered eating in their young adult patients, especially females

  2) How to identify an eating disorder or "disordered eating attitudes and behaviors"

3) How to work with a multidisciplinary team to intervene with the patient and family when a young adult patient with diabetes is struggling with an eating disorder or disordered eating

How to reduce the risk of disordered eating in young adult patients:
- Negotiate realistic blood glucose level, weight, and behavioral goals with patients.
- Avoid perfectionism.
- Allow patients to express their negative feelings about having diabetes. Make it clear that it is normal to occasionally feel burdened by or discouraged with the diabetes regimen.
- Refer to mental health providers if you suspect depression.
- Listen to your patient's concerns about weight and shape.
- Be willing to work with your patients to help them reach realistic weight loss goals.
- All members of the diabetes team should emphasize healthy eating, not dieting. The goal of a diabetes meal plan is flexibility, not restriction. Collaborate with the patient to set realistic weight goals.

How to identify an eating disorder or "disordered eating" in young adult patients:
Some early warning signs of eating disorders may include the following: (Note: These should raise your "index of suspicion" but are not definite signs of an eating disorder.)
- An unexplainable elevated A1C level in a patient knowledgeable about diabetes may indicate the patient is cutting back on insulin to control weight by purging calories from the body through the urine.
- Frequent DKA may be caused by omission of insulin. Patients with serious eating disorders may learn how to avoid hospitalization for DKA by giving themselves only enough insulin to stay out of the hospital.
- Anxiety and avoidance surrounding being weighed may indicate an eating disorder.
- Weight loss or maintenance in the context of self-reported eating patterns that should cause weight gain may indicate that the person is purging calories through insulin omission.

- Bingeing with food or abusing alcohol may occur along with an eating disorder.

Because secrecy is a characteristic of most eating disorders, take the initiative with your patients and ask the following open-ended questions (adapted from Goebel-Fabbri [2002]):
- "How do you feel about your body weight and shape?"
- "How much do you currently weigh? How much would you like to weigh ideally? How often do you weigh yourself?"
- "How do you like your current meal plan? Do you ever feel that it is too difficult to stick to this meal plan or that you are often eating too much or too little?"
- "Do you ever change your insulin dose to influence your weight?"
- "How many shots does your doctor recommend that you take each day, and how many shots do you take on a typical day?"
- "What has your experience been with DKA?"
- "How regular is your menstrual period?"

Antisdel et al. (2001) developed and validated a survey, the Diabetes Eating Problem Survey (DEPS), for detecting symptoms of disordered eating in young women with diabetes. This survey is reprinted in Table 1 with permission from the authors.

TABLE 1. **Survey of Eating Attitudes & Diabetes Management**

Living with diabetes can sometimes be difficult, particularly regarding eating and diabetes management. Listed below are a variety of attitudes and behaviors regarding diabetes management. Please read each item below and circle the number that indicates how often this is true for you <u>over the past four weeks</u>.

0 Never	1 Rarely	2 Sometimes	3 Often	4 Usually	5 Always

1. I check my blood sugar less frequently than my doctor tells me	0	1	2	3	4	5
2. Losing weight is an important goal to me	0	1	2	3	4	5
3. I skip meals and /or snacks	0	1	2	3	4	5
4. Other people have told me that my eating is out of control	0	1	2	3	4	5
5. Before exercising, I eat carbohydrates to avoid going low	0	1	2	3	4	5
6. After I overeat, I don't take enough insulin to cover the food	0	1	2	3	4	5

TABLE 1. Continued

7. I eat more when I am alone than when I am with others	0	1	2	3	4	5
8. I feel that it's difficult to lose weight and control my diabetes at the same time	0	1	2	3	4	5
9. I avoid checking my blood sugar when I feel like it is out of range	0	1	2	3	4	5
10. When my blood sugar is low, I eat something immediately	0	1	2	3	4	5
11. I adjust my insulin dose based on the results of my blood sugar checks	0	1	2	3	4	5
12. I make myself vomit	0	1	2	3	4	5
13. I try to keep my blood sugar high so that I will lose weight	0	1	2	3	4	5
14. I eat in private when no one else is around	0	1	2	3	4	5
15. I try to eat to the point of spilling ketones in my urine	0	1	2	3	4	5
16. I feel fat when I take all of my insulin	0	1	2	3	4	5
17. I forget to take my insulin	0	1	2	3	4	5
18. Other people tell me to take better care of my diabetes	0	1	2	3	4	5
19. After I overeat, I skip my next insulin dose	0	1	2	3	4	5
20. I take less insulin than what my doctor tells me	0	1	2	3	4	5
21. I feel that my eating is out of control	0	1	2	3	4	5
22. I alternate between eating very little and eating huge amounts	0	1	2	3	4	5
23. Controlling my diabetes is very important to me	0	1	2	3	4	5
24. I feel comfortable eating in front of others	0	1	2	3	4	5
25. I would rather be thin than have good control of my diabetes	0	1	2	3	4	5
26. I like to have ketones in my urine because that means that I am burning fat	0	1	2	3	4	5
27. I exercise to control my blood sugars	0	1	2	3	4	5
28. When my blood sugar is high I take extra insulin	0	1	2	3	4	5

How to intervene when you suspect an eating disorder or disordered eating in young adult patients:
- Identify outpatient therapists (psychologists, social workers, psychiatrists) who are not only experienced in treating eating disorders, but also comfortable treating patients with diabetes and an eating disorder.
- Severe eating disorders, especially anorexia nervosa and purging through insulin omission, are life-threatening, and these patients may require hospitalization in an inpatient eating disorders unit. Identify a psychiatric facility that has experience in the treatment of patients with eating disorders and diabetes.
- It is critical that the patient's diabetes team remain in close contact with providers who specialize in the treatment of eating disorders. Multidisciplinary teamwork with close communication is necessary for effective treatment.
- If it is difficult to locate local outpatient or inpatient resources for your patients with diabetes and eating disorders, contact the state medical society, the state diabetes association, IAEDP (International Association of Eating Disorder Professionals), or AABA (American Anorexia and Bulimia Association).

How to minimize weight gain related to intensification of glycemic control:
- Basal/bolus therapy using both glargine and detemir has been shown to be associated with less weight gain than other longer-acting insulins.
- Physiologic basal/bolus insulin replacement more readily facilitates dieting, since mealtime insulin doses can be decreased to adjust for reduced food intake. In addition, with basal/bolus therapy, there is less need for between-meal snacking than with traditional insulin injection regimens.
- With pump therapy, the patient can reduce basal insulin levels during exercise (either by removing the pump or using the "temporary basal" feature), and this will allow him or her to more effectively use exercise to burn off calories without need for carbohydrate loading.

A caution about pump therapy and eating disorders: Sometimes young women with poor glycemic control due to unrecognized eating disorders and insulin omission will be started on the pump with hopes that the technology will help facilitate improved glycemic control. This can be dangerous. Unlike other pump patients who will troubleshoot for insulin nondelivery whenever there is unexplained hyperglycemia, the chronically hyperglycemic individual on a pump will not know when to follow these troubleshooting routines and is therefore more prone to develop ketoacidosis in the event of pump malfunction or catheter occlusion. (A perspective for the patient on diabetes therapy and weight gain, including strategies for weight control during intensification of glycemic control, is presented in More Bumps in the Journey: Intensive Therapy and Weight Gain on page 32.)

D.D.'S STORY

D.D. is a soft-spoken, slim 21-year-old college student, studying to be a nutritionist, who was diagnosed with diabetes when she was 11 years old. She just began seeing an adult endocrinologist who refers her to a mental health professional for depression and poorly controlled diabetes (A1C of 14%). D.D. had previously obtained a prescription for Prozac from her pediatric endocrinologist, but she had run out of medication because she had not seen him in the past four years. D.D. claims that Prozac was helpful for depression and also said that it tended to decrease her blood glucose levels. Even though D.D. had not been seen by her pediatric team for over 4 years, they would refill prescriptions for insulin, but not for Prozac.

D.D. says that she has trouble giving insulin injections, that injections are painful, and that it takes her a long time to complete an insulin injection. Her mental health professional refers her to a CDE to assess her injection technique. The CDE reports that D.D. was using larger-than-needed syringe needles and did show a lot of anxiety when injecting herself. D.D. also had told the CDE that she often skipped shots because she did not have time to inject before her classes in college.

D.D. says that she studies alone every night and that she eats while she studies. She reports bingeing on candy she buys from the campus store or from vending machines in her dorm. She often skips her evening shot and goes to bed feeling exhausted and sick. D.D. finally reveals that she can stay slim, even though she eats a lot of candy, by skipping insulin shots, which are hard for her to do anyway.

Over the next few months, D.D. sees her counselor weekly and learns that she is angry about having diabetes, feels lonely in her family and at college, and is just beginning to grieve for her father who died 5 years ago. When D.D. was first diagnosed, her father gave her insulin injections. Over the next few months, she continues to binge, although less frequently, and begins to take evening insulin more regularly. However, she also begins to gain weight, and with this change in her body, D.D. resumes her habits of skipping evening injections and bingeing. "If I just don't take my nighttime insulin," D.D. says, "I can eat whatever I want, and I lose weight."

D.D.'s adult provider suggested other solutions rather than insulin restriction for losing weight, helping her to learn to safely reduce insulin based on reduced carbohydrate intake and blood glucose monitoring. With this support and repeated medical visits, D.D. slowly learned to adjust insulin based on blood glucose monitoring results and carbohydrate counting to achieve a healthy weight and healthy blood glucose levels.

Set Realistic Blood Glucose Goals

Blood glucose monitoring is a crucial tool in the management of diabetes, and patient glucose records are now a major focus of the patient-provider interaction in diabetes. However, clinicians will often overlook the fact that, for the individual patient, blood glucose and A1C levels are more than just objective measures of glycemic control but also translate into a complex judgment of their performance, competence, and self-worth.

Goal-setting has an important role in the complex process of behavioral change, and the clinician needs to differentiate between recommended clinical treatment standards (such as those outlined in the ADA Clinical Practice Recommendations) and the goals that are set for the individual patient. Giving the patient an *ideal* rather than a *realistic* A1C treatment target can be counterproductive. Goals that are too ambitious and that overlook the realities of the patient's life (for example, the competing priorities faced by the college student) and the complex difficulties of managing diabetes can set the patient up for failure, frustration, and disengagement from care. In contrast, realistic and attainable goals that are appropriate to the patient's aptitude, motivation, and stage of development will reinforce the patient's sense of confidence and self-efficacy, and this will often drive further progress as the goals are further advanced.

Because improved self-care practices underlie improved A1C and blood glucose levels, goal-setting should focus on self-care behavior in addition to biologic targets. Goals need to be set in collaboration with the patient (i.e., *with* rather than *for* the patient), and the patient must be able to relate to the goal at a practical level. For example, patients who are athletic will relate to the importance of optimizing glycemic control around exercise, and this can be a starting point for engaging them to improve their self-care. The suppertime meal will usually vary from day to day, and patients will often relate to the value of adjusting the suppertime insulin dose (just as your pancreas would if you didn't have diabetes) to cover variations in food intake. This can be an entry point for introducing the patient to the concepts of carbohydrate counting and physiologic insulin replacement. New self-care habits need to become an integrated part of daily routines and, to ensure that the patient does not feel overburdened, changes in the diabetes regimen will often need to be introduced gradually.

Having realistic expectations and goals minimizes the risk for frustration and "diabetes burnout." During some of the transitions of the young adult period (such as leaving home, starting college, or starting a new job), even some of the more conscientious patients will have difficulty making their diabetes a high priority. Patients and parents will often need to be reminded that this is usually a "normal" transitory phase and not a sign of personal failure. (A perspective for the patient on goal-setting [Set Attainable Goals on page 36] and glycemic control [Keeping Perspective About Monitoring and Number on page 23] is presented earlier.)

Minimize Performance Pressure About Glycemic Control

Minimizing "performance pressure" about glycemic control can be a key element in reducing burnout and keeping the patient focused on monitoring glucose levels and optimizing diabetes control.

The health care provider can minimize performance pressure by:

- Helping the patient to appreciate that blood glucose monitoring is a tool ("compass") to direct diabetes management rather than a performance measure ("test").
- Individualizing blood glucose and glycohemoglobin targets rather than focusing on an "ideal" and often unattainable "standard."
- Describing glucose and glycohemoglobin levels with neutral language rather than judgmental expressions (for example, "high" or "out of range" instead of "poor" or "bad").

RECOGNIZE THE IMPACT OF CHANGING FAMILY ROLES AND SOCIAL RELATIONSHIPS

The usually abrupt transfer to complete independence and responsibility for self-care that occurs when young adults with diabetes leave home can be unsettling for both them and their parents.

- The developmental maturity of the young adult is an important consideration in deciding when to transfer care from the pediatrician to the adult care provider. Some patients may find the overwhelming changes and demands of the early young adult years a distraction from forging ties with a new physician. The young adult who is facing a difficult adjustment to college and has strong bonds with the pediatric team may do better if the transfer to adult medicine is delayed until after the college years.
- The health care provider needs to be attuned to anxieties that parents may develop as their involvement recedes during their child's passage to independence. Anxious parents who are overly intrusive and controlling can trigger a destructive cycle of "miscarried helping" that undermines their child's self-confidence and motivation.

Josh: A story of "miscarried helping"

Since her son's diagnosis of diabetes when he was 8 years old, Josh's mother had always been aware of all of his blood sugar values. As Josh got older, he was annoyed by his mom checking his meter all the time, but she did not scold or question his out-of-range values; hence,

Josh just let her know all his values. Similarly, she discussed his blood glucose and A1C values with his diabetes doctor and nurse educator at every appointment.

Now that Josh is 19 years old, away in college, and seeing a new adult diabetes provider, his mother feels frantic about his health and worries that he will fail his freshman year at the university. She repeatedly calls his new diabetes team to find out about Josh's blood glucose and A1C values. When she gets no response from his new diabetes doctor, she asks her son to fax home his blood glucose values. Josh refuses and also tells his mother to "back off!" As her anxiety over Josh's health grows, his mother continues to call his new diabetes provider looking for information and reassurance. However, this doctor does not want to break confidentiality with Josh, as a relatively new patient to his practice, or violate the HIPAA (Health Insurance Portability and Accountability Act) guidelines; therefore, the doctor simply never returns his mother's calls. In the meantime, Josh's mother insists that Josh fax his blood sugar values home or she will not pay for his second-semester tuition.

Josh fails to fax his blood sugar logs to his mother. When he returns home at the end of the semester, he meets with his pediatric nurse educator, with whom he has a good rapport. She encourages Josh to give his new diabetes care provider permission to speak with his mother. She mentions to Josh that if his mother is "kept in the loop" about his diabetes, this will lessen her anxieties about him. In turn, Josh's mother has agreed that she will back off.

How to Prevent "Miscarried Helping" and Teach Positive Involvement of Parents of Young Adults

- Encourage the young adult patient to bring a parent for education and updating, *which will be done in the presence of the young adult.*
- Listen to the parent's fears, worries, and experiences with previous diabetes providers. Reassure the parents that your goal is to engage their child in diabetes self-care in a way that will optimize current and future health and to make sure he or she has regular physical and eye exams.

- Emphasize that as a provider you will speak with the parent only when you have the young adult's permission and/or in the presence of both the parent and the young adult patient.
- Model positive helping by directly asking your patient how and when his parents could be of help.
- Especially during the first phase of the young adult period when the young adult is coping with multiple distractions, educate the patient and family to have realistic and appropriate expectations concerning the young adult's blood glucose goals and self-care behaviors.

Helping Guide the Patient in Social Relationships

The health care provider needs to be attuned to how diabetes affects the developing social relationships of the young adult.

- Misunderstandings related to the behavioral changes that occur with unrecognized hypoglycemia are common and can disrupt relationships. Other issues such as unrealistic expectations and blame can sabotage relationships and undermine self-care. Inviting the participation of partners in medical visits can help in uncovering these problems.
- The period when the young adult patient starts to develop permanent relationships and plans for the future will often signal a stage of receptiveness to improving self-care. Life partners can become influential agents for change, and it is often important to engage them in discussions about treatment options and plans.

RECOGNIZE YOUR IMPACT ON THE MENTAL HEALTH OF THE PATIENT

Health care providers have an important role in fostering the mental health of the patient with diabetes. Depression, lack of motivation, and disengagement from self-care can be the unintended consequence of the interactions between the patient and health care professional.

The positive message of the DCCT, and other intervention studies that have established the causal link between glycemic control and the microvascular complications of diabetes, is that individuals have some control over their destiny. However, patients will often perceive another message in this causal link: that they are to blame for their complications. It is often overlooked that, as evidenced by the data showing that some individuals with relatively low A1C levels develop complications, whereas others with poorer control seem to be protected, hyperglycemia is not the only pathogenic factor in the development of complications (Zhang et al. 2001). (Preventing Complications [page 42] presents a perspective for the patient on this issue that may help reduce the cycle of self-blame, despair, and lack of motivation that sometimes develops when complications strike.)

Many patients with diabetes live with a burden of fear and anxiety about complications and disability that will often unwittingly be reinforced by health care professionals. Complications do not escape mention in educational materials on diabetes, and few patients need any reminder of the consequences of neglecting their self-care. There is no evidence that "fear-mongering" is successful in motivating patients. On the contrary, if the interaction with the health professional heightens the patient's fears and anxieties, withdrawal from follow-up and self-care will often result. (Preventing Complications [page 42] presents a perspective that may help reduce the burden of fear and anxiety that is suffered by many patients with diabetes.)

DEVELOPING GUIDELINES

The need to develop guidelines to facilitate the implementation and success of transition programs has been recognized by professional organizations. In 2002, a policy statement by the American Academy of Pediatrics, American Academy of Family Physicians, and the American College of Physicians–American Society of Internal Medicine noted that the goal of an effective transition plan is to provide developmentally appropriate health care services that continue uninterrupted as the individual moves from adolescence to adulthood. Similarly, in 2003, the Society for Adolescent Medicine published a position paper that recognized the vital importance of organized and coordinated transition programs. These position papers offer guidelines for successful transition programs, aimed at facilitating uninterrupted, comprehensive, and accessible care. For example, it is recommended that health care providers partner with the young adult patient, the adult care providers, and the young adult's family. The importance of obtaining ongoing education for all stakeholders (patients, providers, and families) regarding the core knowledge and skills required to provide developmentally appropriate health care transition has been recognized. Written transition plans, completed in collaboration with adolescents aged 14 and older and their families, should be developed and should include information regarding the specific health services needed, who will provide them, and how they will be financed. This plan should be reviewed and updated annually and should include discussions regarding continuous health care insurance coverage that should consider the costs of transition planning and care coordination. Finally, the position papers recognized the need for collaborative development of "best practices" for the management of adults with diseases of childhood (American Academy of Pediatrics 2002, Society for Adolescent Medicine 2003).

The special needs of the emerging adult with diabetes fall outside the focus of the current health care system. Epidemiology studies show that a subset of the young adult population with diabetes is at high risk for accelerated microvascular complications and death from acute metabolic decompensation, and that psychosocial issues are a major underlying risk factor. Furthermore, follow-up data from the DCCT indicate that intensive treatment during adolescence does not necessarily set the stage for optimal glucose control during young adulthood. These findings underscore the importance of considering behavioral and developmental issues in the evaluation and care of the young adult patient with diabetes.

The needs of emerging adults require a multifaceted program, aimed at addressing the needs of this particularly vulnerable and important population of individuals living with diabetes. A number of important organizations have put forward recommendations regarding the development of transition plans for individuals leaving their pediatric providers and moving toward adult care providers. Our review of the existing literature suggests that the evidence base guiding the clinical care of the young adult with diabetes is limited. Based on our clinical experiences and our review of the existing literature, we put forth a set of recommendations (Weissberg-Benchell et al. 2007) to help pediatric and adult providers care for the needs of those transitioning to adult care.

Postlude: Looking Ahead

As mentioned in the Prelude to this book, we have written this guide based on our collective clinical experiences with youth with diabetes and their families. These individuals have taught us about the complexities of the journey for youth and their parents who are maturing across "emerging adulthood" with type 1 diabetes. Clearly, there is a great need for empirical research on the efficacy and effectiveness of different transition plans between pediatric diabetes clinicians and adult diabetes care providers. However, until there is a clear evidence base of strategies for delivering care to young adults with diabetes and their families, we hope that the clinical guidelines presented here will provide assistance to young adults, their families, and diabetes clinicians in this journey.

Bibliography

ACE Inhibitors in Diabetic Nephropathy Trialist Group. Should all patients with type 1 diabetes mellitus and microalbuminuria receive angiotensin-converting enzyme inhibitors? A meta-analysis of individual patient data. *Ann Intern Med* 134:370–379, 2001

American Academy of Pediatrics, American Academy of Family Physicians, American College of Physicians–American Society of Internal Medicine. A consensus statement on health care transitions for young adults with special health care needs. *Pediatrics* 110:1304–1306, 2002

American Diabetes Association. Preventative foot care in people with diabetes. *Diabetes Care* 26(Suppl.1):S78–S79, 2002

———. Preconception care of women with diabetes. *Diabetes Care* 26 (Suppl. 1):S91–S93, 2003

———. Physical activity/exercise and diabetes. *Diabetes Care* 27 (Suppl. 1):S58–S62, 2004

———. Standards of medical care in diabetes. *Diabetes Care* 31 (Suppl. 1):S12–S54, 2008

———. *Complete Guide to Diabetes.* 4th ed. Alexandria, VA, American Diabetes Association, 2005

American Psychiatric Association. *Diagnostic and Statistical Manual of Mental Disorders.* 4th ed. Text Revision (DSM IV-TR). Washington, DC, American Psychiatric Association, 2000

Anderson B. Personal communication, Houston, TX, 2008

Anderson R, Funnell M. *The Art of Empowerment: Stories and Strategies for Diabetes Educators.* Alexandria, VA, American Diabetes Association, 2000

Antisdel JE, Laffel L, Anderson BJ. Improved detection of eating problems in women with type 1 diabetes using a newly developed survey (Abstract). *Diabetes* 50 (Suppl. 1):A47, 2001

Arnett JJ. Emerging adulthood: a theory of development from the late teens through the twenties. *Am Psychol* 55:469–480, 2000

————. *Emerging Adulthood: The Winding Road from the Late Teens through the Twenties.* New York, Oxford University Press, 2004

Barber B, Harmon E. Violating the self: parental psychological control of children and adolescents. In *Intrusive Parenting: How Psychological Control Affects Children and Adolescents.* Washington, DC, American Psychological Association, p. 15–52, 2002

Betz CL, Telfair J. Health care transitions: an introduction. In *Promoting Health Care Transitions for Adolescents with Special Health Care Needs and Disabilities.* Betz CL, Nehring WM, Eds. Baltimore, MD, Paul H. Brookes, p. 3–19, 2007

Bjornsen KD. Health care transition in congenital heart disease: the providers' view point. *Nurs Clin North Am* 39:715–726, 2004

Brumfield K, Lansbury G. Experiences of adolescents with cystic fibrosis during their transition from paediatric to adult health care: a qualitative study of young Australian adults. *Disabil Rehabil* 26:223–234, 2004

Bryden KS, Dunger DB, Mayou RA, Peveler RC, Neil HA. Poor prognosis of young adults with type 1 diabetes: a longitudinal study. *Diabetes Care* 26:1052–1057, 2003

Bryden KS, Neil A, Mayou RA, Peveler RC, Fairburn CG, Dunger DB. Eating habits, body weight, and insulin misuse: a longitudinal study of teenagers and young adults with type 1 diabetes. *Diabetes Care* 22:1956–1960, 1999

Bryden KS, Peveler RC, Stein A, Neil A, Mayou RA, Dunger DB. Clinical and psychological course of diabetes from adolescence to young adulthood. *Diabetes Care* 24:1536–1540, 2001

Dahlquist G, Källen B. Mortality in childhood-onset type 1 diabetes. *Diabetes Care* 28:2384–2387, 2005

Diabetes Control and Complications Trial Research Group. The relationship of glycemic exposure to the risk of development and progression of retinopathy in the Diabetes Control and Complications Trial. *Diabetes* 44:968–983, 1995

Diabetes Control and Complications Trial/Epidemiology of Diabetes Interventions and Complications Research Group. Retinopathy and nephropathy in patients with type 1 diabetes four years after a trial of intensive therapy. *N Engl J Med* 342:381–389, 2000

———. Beneficial effects of intensive therapy during adolescence: outcomes after the conclusion of the Diabetes Control and Complications Trial. *J Pediatr* 139:804–812, 2001

Dovey-Pearce G, Hurrell R, May C, Walker C, Doherty Y. Young adults' (16–25 years) suggestions for providing developmentally appropriate diabetes services: a qualitative study. *Health and Social Care in the Community* 13:409–419, 2005

Eccles JS, Miller-Buchanan C, Flanagan C, Fuligni A, Midgley C, Yee D. Control versus autonomy during adolescence. *J Soc Issues* 47:53–68, 1991

Eiser C, Flynn M, Green E, Havermans T, Kirby R, Sandeman D, Tooke JE. Coming of age with diabetes: patients' views of a clinic for under-25 year olds. *Diabet Med* 10:285–289, 1993

El-Hashimy M, Angelico MC, Martin BC, Krolewski AS, Warram JH. Factors modifying the risk of IDDM in offspring of an IDDM parent. *Diabetes* 44:295–299, 1995

Erikson EH. *Childhood and Society.* New York, Norton, 1950

———. *Identity, Youth and Crisis.* New York, Norton, 1968

Freed GL, Hudson EJ. Transitioning children with chronic diseases to adult care: current knowledge, practices, and directions. *J Pediatr* 148:824–827, 2006

Gallen I. Exercise and type 1 diabetes. *Diabet Med* 20:2–5, 2003

———. Diabetes and sport: managing the complex interactions. *Br J Hosp Med* 67:512–515, 2006

Gillibrand R, Stevenson J. The extended health belief model applied to the experience of diabetes in young people. *Br J Health Psychol* 11:155–169, 2006

Goebel-Fabbri A. Detecting and treating eating disorders in young women with type 1 diabetes. In *Practical Psychology for Diabetes Clinicians.* 2nd ed. Anderson BJ, Rubin RR, Eds. Alexandria, VA, American Diabetes Association, 2002, p. 239–247

Goebel-Fabbri A, Fikkan J, Franko DL, Pearson K, Anderson BJ, Weinger K. Insulin restriction and associated morbidity and mortality in women with type 1 diabetes. *Diabetes Care* 31:415–419, 2008

Hauser ST, Jacobson AM, Lavori P, Wolfsdorf JI, Herskowitz RD, Milley JE, Bliss R, Wertlieb D, Stein J. Adherence among children and adolescents with insulin-dependent diabetes mellitus over a 4-year longitudinal follow-up: immediate and long-term linkages with the family milieu. *J Pediatr Psychol* 15:527–542, 1990

Henricsson M, Nyström L, Blohmé G, Ostman J, Kullberg C, Svensson M, Schölin A, Arnqvist HJ, Björk E, Bolinder J, Eriksson JW, Sundkvist G. The incidence of retinopathy 10 years after diagnosis in young adult people with diabetes. *Diabetes Care* 26:349–354, 2003

Holmbeck GN, Coakley RM, Hommeyer JS, Shapera WE, Westhoven VC. Observed and perceived dyadic and systemic functioning in families of preadolescents with spina bifida. *J Pediatr Psychol* 27:177–189, 2002

Hovind P, Tarnow L, Rossing K, Rossing P, Eising S, Larsen N, Binder C, Parving H-H. Decreasing incidence of severe diabetic microangiopathy in type 1 diabetes. *Diabetes Care* 26:1258–1264, 2003

Jacobson A, Hauser S, Powers S, Noam G. Ego development in diabetic adolescents. *Pediatr Adol Endocrin* 10:1–8, 1982

Jimenez CC, Corcoran MH, Crawley J, Hornsby WG, Peer KS, Philbin RD, Riddell MC. National Athletic Trainers' Association Position Statement: Management of the athlete with type 1 diabetes mellitus. *J Athl Train* 42:536–545, 2007

Jones JM, Lawson MI, Daneman D, Olmsted MP, Rodin G. Eating disorders in adolescent females with and without diabetes. *Br Med J* 320:1563–1566, 2000

Kipps S, Bahu T, Ong K, Acklandt FM, Brown RS, Fox CT, Griffin NK, Knight AH, Mann NP, Neil HW, Simpson H, Edge JA, Dunger DB. Current methods of transfer of young people with type 1 diabetes to adult services. *Diabet Med* 19:649–654, 2002

Kokkonen J, Lautala P, Salmela P. The state of young adults with juvenile onset diabetes. *Int J Circumpolar Health* 56:76–85, 1997

———. Social maturation in juvenile onset diabetes. *Acta Paediatr* 83:279–284, 1994

Krolewski AS, Warram JH, Christlieb AR, Busick EJ, Kahn CR. The changing natural history of nephropathy in type 1 diabetes. *Am J Med* 78:785–794, 1985

Lachin JM, Genuth S, Nathan DM, Zinman B, Rutledge BN. Effect of glycemic exposure on the risk of microvascular complications in the Diabetes Control and Complications Trial—revisited. *Diabetes* 57:995–1001, 2008

Laing SP, Swerdlow AJ, Slater SD, Botha JL, Burden AC, Waugh NR, Smith AW, Hill RD, Bingley PJ, Patterson CC, Qiao Z, Keen H. The British Diabetic Association Cohort Study, I: All-cause mortality in patients with insulin-treated diabetes mellitus. *Diabet Med* 16:459–465, 1999a

———. The British Diabetic Association Cohort Study, II: Cause-specific mortality in patients with insulin-treated diabetes mellitus. *Diabet Med* 16:466–471, 1999b

Laing SP, Jones ME, Swerdlow AJ, Burden AC, Gatling W. Psychosocial and socioeconomic risk factors for premature death in young people with diabetes. *Diabetes Care* 28:1618–1623, 2005

Levinson DJ, Darrow CN, Klein EB, et al. *The Seasons of Man's Life.* New York, Knopf, 1978

Litt AS. *The College Student's Guide to Eating Well on Campus.* Bethesda, MD, Tulip Hill Press, 2000

LoCasale-Crouch J, Johnson B. Transition from pediatric to adult medical care: *Adv Chronic Kidney Dis* 12:412–417, 2005

Lorenzen T, Pociot F, Stilgren L, Kristiansen OP, Johannesen J, Olsen PB, Walmar A, Larsen A, Albrechtsen NC, Eskildsen PC, Andersen OO, Nerup J. Predictors of IDDM recurrence in offspring of Danish IDDM patients. *Diabetologia* 41:666–673, 1998

Lotstein DS, McPherson M, Strickland B, Newacheck PW. Transition planning for youth with special health care needs: results from the national survey of children with special health care needs. *Pediatrics* 115:1562–1568, 2005

Lustman PJ, Singh PK, Clouse RE. Recognizing and managing depression in patients with diabetes. In *Practical Psychology for Diabetes Clinicians.* 2nd ed. Anderson BJ, Rubin RR, Eds. Alexandria, VA, American Diabetes Association, 2002, p. 229–238

Maguire AM, Craig ME, Craighead A. Autonomic nerve testing predicts the development of complications. *Diabetes Care* 30:77–82, 2007

Mathiesen ER, Hommel E, Hansen HP, Schmidt UM, Parving H-H. Randomised controlled trial of long-term efficacy of captopril on preservation of kidney function in normotensive patients with insulin-dependent diabetes and microalbuminuria. *Br Med J* 319:24–25, 1999

McDonagh JE, Southwood TR, Shaw KL. Unmet education and training needs of rheumatology health professionals in adolescent health and transitional care. *Rheumatology* 43:737–743, 2004

Mellinger DC. Preparing students with diabetes for life at college. *Diabetes Care* 26:2675–2678, 2003

Myers J. Transition into adulthood with a chronic illness focus: insulin-dependent diabetes mellitus. *Dissertation Abstracts International* 53:3182, 1997

Nathan DM, Kuenen J, Borg R, Zheng H, Schoenfeld D, Heine RJ. Translating the A1C assay into estimated average glucose. *Diabetes Care* 31:1–6, 2008

Pacaud D, McConnell B, Huot C, Aebi C, Yale JF. Transition from pediatric to adult care for insulin-dependent diabetes patients. *Can J Diabetes* 20:13–20, 1996

Pacaud D, Yale JF, Stephure D, Trussell, R, Dele-Davies H. Problems in transition from pediatric care to adult care for individuals with diabetes. *Can J Diabetes* 29:13–18, 2005

Pacaud D, Crawford S, Stephure DK, Dean HJ, Couch R, Dewey D. Effect of type 1 diabetes on psychosocial maturation in young adults. *J Adolesc Health* 40:29–35, 2007

Perkins BA, Ficociello LH, Silva KH, Finkelstein DM, Warram JH, Krolewski AS. Regression of microalbuminuria in type 1 diabetes. *N Engl J Med* 348:2285–2293, 2003

Peveler RC, Bryden KS, Neil HAW, Fairburn CG, Mayou RA, Dunger DB, Turner HM. The relationship of disordered eating habits and attitudes to clinical outcome in young adult females with type 1 diabetes. *Diabetes Care* 28:84–88, 2005

Peyrot M, Aanstoot H-J, for DAWN Youth Survey Group. Sources of support associated with patient and parent behavioral/psychosocial outcomes in the multi-national DAWN Youth Survey. *Diabetes* 57 (Suppl. 1):36A, 2008

Polonsky WH, Anderson BJ, Lohrer P, Aponte JE, Jacobson AM, Cole CF. Insulin omission in women with IDDM. *Diabetes Care* 17:1178–1185, 1994

Robinson N, Yateman NA, Protopapa LE, Bush L. Unemployment and diabetes. *Diabet Med* 6:797–803, 1989

Ruderman N, Devlin JT, Schneider SH, Kriska A (Eds.). *Handbook of Exercise in Diabetes*. Alexandria, VA, American Diabetes Association, 2002

Rydall AC, Rodin GM, Olmsted MP, Devenyi RG, Daneman D. Disordered eating behavior and microvascular complications in young women with insulin-dependent diabetes mellitus. *N Engl J Med* 336:1849–1854, 1997

Scal P, Evans T, Blozis S, Okinow N, Blum R. Trends in transition from pediatric to adult health care services for young adults with chronic conditions. *J Adolesc Health* 24:259–264, 1999

Scal P, Ireland M. Addressing transition to adult health care for adolescents with special health care needs. *Pediatrics* 115:1607–1612, 2005

Seiffge-Krenke I. *Diabetic Adolescents and Their Families: Stress, Coping, and Adaptation.* New York City, NY, Cambridge University Press, 2001

Shaw KL, Southwood TR, McDonagh JE. Developing a programme of transitional care for adolescents with juvenile idiopathic arthritis: results of a postal survey. *Rheumatology* 43:211–219, 2004

Skrivarhaug T, Bangstad H-J, Stene LC, Sandvik L, Hanssen KF, Joner G. Long-term mortality in a nationwide cohort of childhood-onset type 1 diabetic patients in Norway. *Diabetologia* 49:298–305, 2006

Society for Adolescent Medicine. Transition to adult care for adolescent and young adults with chronic conditions. *Adolescent Health* 33:309–311, 2003

Stabile L, Rosser L, Porterfield KM, McCauley S, Levenson C, Haglund J, Christman K. Transfer versus transition: success in pediatric transplantation brings the welcome challenge of transition. *Prog Transplant* 15:363–370, 2005

Steinberg L. Interdependency in the family: autonomy, conflict, and harmony. In *At the Threshold: The Developing Adolescent.* Feldman S, Eliot G, Eds. Cambridge, MA, Harvard University Press, 1990

Svensson M, Sundkvist G, Arnqvist HJ, Björk E, Blohmé G, Bolinder J, Henricsson M, Nyström L, Torffvit O, Waernbaum I, Ostman J, Eriksson JM. Signs of nephropathy may occur early in young adults with diabetes despite modern diabetes management. *Diabetes Care* 26:2903–2909, 2003

Telfair J, Alexander LR, Loosier PS, Alleman-Velez PL, Simmons J. Providers' perspectives and beliefs regarding transition to adult care for adolescents with sickle cell disease. *J Health Care Poor Underserved* 15:443–461, 2004

Thompson CJ, Cumming JF, Chalmers J, Gould C, Newton RW. How have patients reacted to the implications of the DCCT? *Diabetes Care* 19:876–879, 1996

U.K. Prospective Diabetes Study Group. Tight blood pressure control and risk of macrovascular and microvascular complications in type 2 diabetes: UKPDS 38. *Br Med J* 317:703–713, 1998

Van Walleghem N, MacDonald CA, Dean HJ. Building connections for young adults with type 1 diabetes mellitus in Manitoba: feasibility and acceptability of a transition initiative. *Chronic Dis Can* 27:130–134, 2006

Vinicor F. Barriers to translation of the Diabetes Control and Complications Trial. *Diabetes Rev* 2:371–383, 1994

Visentin K, Koch T, Kralik D. Adolescents with type 1 diabetes: transition between diabetes services. *J Clin Nurs* 15:761–769, 2006

Wadwa RP, Kinney GL, Maahs DM, Snell-Bergeon J, Hokanson JE, Garg SK, Eckel RH, Rewers M. Awareness and treatment of dyslipidemia in young adults with type 1 diabetes. *Diabetes Care* 28:1051–1056, 2005

Waernbaum I, Blohmé G, Ostman J, Sundkvist G, Eriksson JW, Arnqvist HJ, Bolinder J, Nyström L. Excess mortality in incident cases of diabetes mellitus aged 15 to 34 years at diagnosis: a population-based study (DISS) in Sweden. *Diabetologia* 49:653–659, 2006

Warram JH, Martin BC, Krolewski AS. Risk of IDDM in children of diabetic mothers decreases with increasing maternal age at pregnancy. *Diabetes* 40:1679–1684, 1991

Wdowik MJ, Kendall PA, Harris MA. College students with diabetes: using focus group and interviews to determine psychosocial issues and barriers to control. *Diabetes Educator* 23:558–562, 1997

Weissberg-Benchell J, Wolpert H, Anderson B. Transitioning from pediatric to adult care: a new approach to the post-adolescent young person with type 1 diabetes. *Diabetes Care* 30:2441–2446, 2007

Welch GW, Jacobson A, Polonsky WH. The Problem Areas in Diabetes (PAID) Scale: An examination of its clinical utility. *Diabetes Care* 20:760–766, 1997

Wibell L, Nyström L, Ostman J, Arnqvist H, Blohmé G, Lithner F, Littorin B, Sundkvist G. Increased mortality in diabetes during the first 10 years of the disease: a population-based study (DISS) in Swedish adults 15–34 years old at diagnosis. *J Intern Med* 249:263–270, 2001

Wolpert H (Ed.). *Smart Pumping for People with Diabetes: A Practical Approach to Mastering the Insulin Pump.* Alexandria, VA, American Diabetes Association, 2002

Wolpert HA, Anderson BJ. Young adults with diabetes: need for a new treatment paradigm. *Diabetes Care* 24:1514–1514, 2001

Wysocki T, Hough BS, Ward KM, Green LB. Diabetes mellitus in the transition to adulthood: adjustment, self-care, and health status. *J Dev Behav Pediatr* 13:194–201, 1992

Zhang L, Krzentowski G, Albert A, Lefebvre PJ. Risk of developing retinopathy in Diabetes Control and Complications Trial type 1 diabetic patients with good or poor metabolic control. *Diabetes Care* 24:1275–1279, 2001

Index

A

ACE inhibitors, 44, 45
A1C levels
  CGM and, 27
  complications and, 8, 42–43, 73,
    79, 84, 98
  perceptions of, 93–94
  in pregnancy, 51
  ADA guidelines, 57, 79
  Adherence issues
  behavioral problems in, 6–8, 73
  eating disorders and, 87
  provider's approach to, 82–83
  support and, 7
Adrenaline (epinephrine), 55, 57
Adulthood, attributes of, 4
Advocate/educator role, 61, 64
Alarm burnout, 32
Alcohol
  as calorie source, 34, 53
  eating disorders and, 88
  glucose control and, 22

hyperglycemia and, 53
as hypoglycemia cause, 25,
  52–54, 77
mortality from, 72
Amputations, 45–46
Anderson, R., 82–83
Anorexia, 87, 91
Antidepressants, 76, 92
Apidra, 17
Arnett, J.J., 3–4, 7
Aspart, 19

B

Basal/bolus therapy, 19, 26, 35, 91
Behavioral issues
  ADA guidelines, 79
  in adherence, 6–8, 73
  changes, reinforcement of, 79
  evaluation of, 79–80
  glycemic control and, 6–8, 12, 73
  predictors of, 6–7, 9
Beta-cells, pancreatic, 17
Binge eating, 88, 93

Other Titles from the
American Diabetes Association

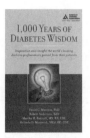

1,000 Years of Diabetes Wisdom
edited by David G. Marrero, PhD; Robert Anderson, EdD; Martha M. Funnell, MS, RN, CDE; and Melinda D. Maryniuk, MEd, RD, CDE
This anthology of more than 50 stories focuses on the other side of treating diabetes—what providers can learn from their patients. With more than 1,000 combined years of patient-care experience, the contributors share their knowledge and foresight and the life-altering experiences that both challenge and change the way care providers care for their patients.
Order no. 5435-01; Price $19.95

Diabetes 911: How to Handle Everyday Emergencies
by Larry A. Fox, MD, and Sandra L. Weber, MD
When it comes to a condition as serious as diabetes, the best way to solve problems is to prevent them from ever happening. Do you know what to do in case of an emergency? With *Diabetes 911,* you will learn the necessary skills to handle hypoglycemia, insulin pump malfunctions, natural disasters, travel, depression, and sick days.
Order no. 4887-01; Price $12.95

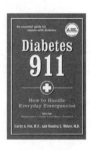

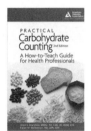

Practical Carbohydrate Counting, 2nd ed.
by Hope S. Warshaw, MMSc, RD, CDE, BC-ADM, and Karen M. Bolderman, RD, LDN, CDE
The essentials of teaching carbohydrate counting are presented in this revised and much expanded edition. This resource provides clear and practical approaches that will allow you to help yor patients achieve glycemic control with Basic or Advanced Carbohydrate Counting.
Order no. 5619-02; Price $22.95

Smart Pumping
edited by Howard Wolpert, MD
Smart Pumping integrates the technology of insulin pumps with the physical and psychological aspects of diabetes care. It provides a comprehensive approach toward diabetes management and pump therapy with an honest appreciation of the real-life challenges and frustrations pumpers face every day.
Order no. 4835-01; Price $16.95

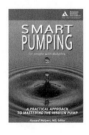

Order this and other American Diabetes Association books and resources
for health care professionals at **http://store.diabetes.org**
or by calling **1-800-232-6733**.